Breathe Easy

Simple Ways to Stay Well Connected

By

Braith Bamkin

Cover design: Nicki Averill

Typesetting: Clockwork Graphic Design

Printing: Printed in Australia by Ovato Print Pty Ltd

Published by Peritia Press

Contents

Introduction

Have you ever been introduced to something that you know is going to be really good for you, yet from the outside it seems as though it's just another thing to add to your 'to do' list?

Conscious breathing can seem quite inaccessible to a lot of people. Not everyone relates to the pathway of Eastern spirituality that conscious breathing brings to mind, or to the complex and sometimes confusing methods that have been popularised by some modern Western breath work practitioners.

However, it is entirely possible to take the traditions and techniques of breath work and apply them in simple and effective ways, in a business context and in your personal life.

My interest in conscious breathing started over thirty years ago, when I began practicing yoga and meditation. Many yoga teachers talk about breath and breathing, and incorporate this into their classes, although it is often not presented in a way that is readily understood, as the use of Sanskrit terms creates a barrier for many people, and teachers rarely explain the 'how', and, more importantly, the 'why'.

The greatest association that conscious breathing has in many people's minds is in relation to mindfulness. Although there is an increasing awareness of the importance and benefits of mindfulness in promoting wellbeing, understanding how to incorporate the practice into daily life can feel confusing. I am often asked what 'being mindful' means, and how mindfulness can be practised.

In recent years, there has been a shift from the traditional Eastern roots of conscious breathing, with the principles gaining popularity in Western culture. Even in this context, the methods that have been put forward can require prolonged study. Once again, this can leave conscious breathing feeling very inaccessible, particularly for business people facing time pressures in their busy professional and personal lives.

The good news is that it doesn't need to be like this. I have been successfully applying conscious breathing techniques in numerous business situations for many years. Although I am a practitioner of yoga and meditation, the foundation of the techniques I use are rooted in science, rather than spiritual practices, and the ways in which these techniques can be applied are straightforward and accessible to all.

The purpose of writing this book is to bring the concept of conscious breathing into a format that enables professionals like you to gain the benefit of a practice that has been around for thousands of years, in a way that is relevant and appropriate in the context of a contemporary lifestyle.

The pressures of the modern work environment are numerous, and include everything from physical problems such as neck, shoulder, and back pain, psychological problems such as stress and anxiety, interpersonal problems such as workplace conflicts, and staff problems, such as lack of engagement.

Breathe Easy: Simple Ways to Stay Well Connected is a well-grounded and practical way of using conscious breathing to enhance your business life and improve your workplace environment in a way that counteracts these problems.

As Executive Director for a successful BNI region in Melbourne, Australia[1], I am in the privileged position of being able to observe the traits of those business owners and entrepreneurs who are very successful. I have learned that successful people have the ability to be present and to connect deeply with those around them. Conscious breathing and laughter yoga are tools that I use, and that I see help achieve these states for business success.

Breathe Easy: Simple Ways to Stay Well Connected guides you through:

- The mechanics of breathing, to enable you to improve energy, focus, and concentration, and to minimise stress, anxiety, and feelings of overwhelm.

- Different techniques to energise, balance, and calm you, in order to get the most out of

[1]BNI is the world's largest professional referral organisation, with hundreds of thousands of members across seventy plus countries, who generate billions of dollars of referrals for each other every year. For further information on BNI see www.bnimc.com.au for my Melbourne region or www.bni.com if you are outside Melbourne.

meetings, presentations, and negotiations, as well as helping to manage the day-to-day demands of your working life.

- The importance of ergonomics and posture in enhancing physical wellbeing and generating positive energy flow between the body and the brain.

- The principles of Behavioural Activation, and how you can use conscious breathing to change your state of being.

Packed full of exercises, examples, tips and techniques, *Breathe Easy: Simple Ways to Stay Well Connected* gives you a detailed insight into how you can apply conscious breathing in a working environment, in order to benefit every aspect of your professional life.

Important Notice

Everything I teach is designed to be simple, so that it does not have any negative impact on your health. If any of the practices in this book create feelings of discomfort, light-headedness, dizziness, or pain, stop immediately, and breathe slowly and calmly, in a seated position.

Never practice any breathing techniques in water, especially when you are by yourself. This includes baths, pools, rivers, and the ocean. Never practice energising or calming breathing techniques whilst operating machinery or driving.

Conscious breathing is not an endurance sport. There are no prizes for coming first. It is not a competition.

Breathe sensibly, and enjoy. If it's not fun, then stop.

Chapter One

Coming Up For Air

Why Explore Conscious Breathing?

As a busy professional, your ability to juggle numerous tasks and roles is exceptional. You're ticking all the boxes and hitting all the targets. Creating space for anything else in your world is only going to happen if it adds value. It is for this reason that conscious breathing is such an exceptional tool.

When you practice conscious breathing, you don't need to create space to incorporate something new. The opposite is true. Conscious breathing gives you greater clarity of thought, higher levels of energy, and deeper relaxation, and so the practice actually creates *more* space in your life.

There are aspects of the science behind conscious breathing that it is helpful to understand. The exercises that I use, and share in this book, are straightforward. By making a few simple adjustments to something that you do 24/7, you can make great improvements across numerous different areas of your professional and personal life, from managing conflict, to creating abundance and business success, to enhancing fulfilling personal relationships, at work and at home.

Conscious breathing does not add to your 'to do' list. It just makes it easier to work through the tasks.

All the systems of your body perform their functions automatically. You do not, and cannot, consciously control the circulation of your blood, the absorption of nutrients, or the processing of information from your senses.

There is one notable exception to this inability to consciously control your body's systems, and that is breathing. Your respiratory system is the only system in your body that you can take control of and, by doing so, create an immediate, positive effect.

Changing the pattern of your breathing can bring you up when you're down, bring you down when you're up, and balance you throughout the day. Awareness of your breathing can manage your mood and adjust your entire outlook more effectively than any legal (or illegal) drug available. This is the essence of conscious breathing.

Everyone Knows How To Breathe

With so many things to think about, why focus on something that happens naturally?

Of course it is true that breathing will take place unconsciously, without you needing to give it any thought. If you don't breathe, quite simply, you'll die. However, there is a difference between doing something, and doing it well. Many people think that because breathing happens naturally it doesn't need to become the focus of attention. Conscious breathing can and will improve the quality of your life.

The reality is that the world throws us a lot of challenges. At this period in history those challenges are coming at a rate of knots, and things are changing really fast. I started writing this book just before Covid-19 shut the world down. Using conscious breathing techniques helped me, and those that I teach, to navigate this one-in-a-hundred-year challenge.

Change is inevitable. It's how we navigate change that will determine the success of our lives. The modern lifestyle changes rapidly, yet our bodies are not keeping up with these external changes, and many of us are reacting physically to these environmental changes in negative ways.

The demands of our business lives mean that we are now hunched over computers for hours and hours every day, and many of us are working from home in an environment that was never designed to be the primary place of business. We're in one high-pressure meeting after another, often using online formats that further disconnect us from those around us. We're asked to do more, in a competitive global market, and study after study shows that our stress levels are continuing to rise. The future is slowly killing many of us, without us even knowing.

Technology was supposed to make our lives easier and reduce the number of hours that we worked. In fact, we are working longer hours under more pressure. The thinking is that 'more, more, more' is 'better, better, better'. Somehow, working longer and harder has become a badge of honour for many people.

To add to this pressure, the workplace has changed. Going back just a couple of generations, the expectation was that you finished school, got a job, and stayed with that company for the rest of your working life.

Job security is no longer a given. The casualisation of the workforce, coupled with the increasing number of people turning to entrepreneurship, has created levels of stress that people have never had to face before. Where there was security, we now live with uncertainty as a constant, and unwelcome, companion. The consequences of this affect our mental and physical health.

Covid-19 rapidly expanded the working-from-home culture. Sitting for hours and hours on chairs that have not been ergonomically designed, at desks that are rarely the correct height, with lighting that is often poor, all impacts on the ease of our breath, and in many cases constricts proper breathing. The physical tension that your body carries as a result of this constriction then creates mental tension and anxiety.

The way we work isn't going to change any time soon, and so we need to take ownership of our physical and mental wellbeing. The fastest way to achieve this is through the breath.

The common use of phrases such as 'breathe through it', 'just breathe', and 'take a deep breath' show that at a very fundamental level we know that focusing on our breathing is crucial to our wellbeing. From moments of shock and stress through to panic attacks, we recognise the importance of breathing. Conscious breathing transforms our instinctive understanding into a valuable tool. Our body knows what we need, we just get in its way sometimes.

Just Breathe

Conscious breathing gives you the opportunity to connect to yourself. It gives you control, so that you can create your desired state.

When you're concentrating on your breathing, your monkey mind, which generates the constant chatter and negative self-talk, can start to let go. If you're fully focused on breathing, it's hard to have another thought coming in.

In essence, conscious breathing is a very quick, simple, easy route into being present. All the equipment you need is in-built, you can do it wherever you are, it is accessible to everyone, and with a basic understanding of the techniques, it is completely safe.

You can use conscious breathing without anyone being aware of what you are doing, in situations ranging from speaking to clients, colleagues, and teams, during meetings, or while giving speeches and presentations.

For all of these reasons, and many more that we shall explore throughout this book, conscious breathing can have an extremely positive impact on your life, and on the lives of everyone around you.

Exercise – Breath Test

For this exercise, you will need a stopwatch (such as a clock, a watch, or the timer on your phone), a pen, and a piece of paper.

Using your stopwatch, sit upright in a chair and count the number of breaths you take in one minute. It's important that you don't change your normal pattern of breathing in any way when you do this exercise. The aim is to get a better understanding of how you naturally breathe.

If you are finding it difficult not to change the speed or pattern of your breathing because you have now focused your attention on it, then wait five minutes until you are breathing without thinking about it, and then try again.

Once you have measured the number of breaths you are taking in a minute, you have a baseline for your breathing.

Once you have your baseline, stand in front of a mirror and make a note of:

- the number of breaths you are taking
- whether you are breathing through your nose or your mouth
- whether or not you can see your abdomen moving in and out

- whether or not you can see your ribs moving
- whether or not you can see your shoulders moving.

Repeat side-on.

Once you have observed and made a note of all these points, you will have an overview of your pattern of breathing.

Bad Breath

At around the age of five and a half we start to breathe in an unnatural way, as the world around us begins to impact on the way we breathe.

Once we stop running around and playing freely, and begin going to school, where we sit for hours on end at a desk, and spend increasing amounts of time on electronic devices, bad habits start to form. This is when people begin to breathe in a vertical, rather than a horizontal, fashion, which will be discussed in more detail later. As Dr Belisa Vranich discusses in her book, '*Breathe*', "It is anatomically incongruous and biomechanically unsound for us to breathe this way." In spite of how unnatural it is to breathe in this way, many people form these habits, and often don't even realise they've created them.

Societal expectations further impact our breathing. For example, there is a belief that yawning is a sign of rudeness. From a young age we are told that if we yawn we are displaying a lack of interest. In fact, yawning is simply our body needing to take in more air, as discussed by Dan Brulé in his book, *Just Breathe*.

Our society is obsessed with flat stomachs. Just look at any young social media influencer for evidence of this. However, the human body is designed to breathe horizontally, which necessitates breathing into the abdomen so that the belly expands, and the rib cage broadens in a circular fashion.

Think about what happens when you experience shock or fright. You naturally brace your abdomen and your core, because you are preparing for attack. This is a logical thing to do, as by holding everything in really tightly so that your muscles are tense, you are less physically vulnerable. The problem is that when you are not in a fight or flight situation and you hold your core in tension, your brain still receives the message that you are in danger and keeps your stress levels elevated.

The desire to appear thin means that many people are afraid to breathe from their abdomen, and instead hold their core really tightly. In addition, they often wear clothes that are too tight, and this restriction sends a constant message to the brain that creates a muscular and emotional corset around the middle of the body. Later in this book we will practice some exercises to help you gain awareness of this and assist in liberating you from this pressure.

Breathing Inhibitors Checklist

All of the points on this checklist can negatively impact your ability to breathe correctly.

- Sitting in front of a computer for prolonged periods of time
- Playing computer games for hours on end

- Sitting in a car for prolonged periods of time
- Wearing tight or restrictive clothing
- Childhood anxiety and trauma
- Frequent texting – known as 'tech neck'
- Carrying heavy bags and equipment
- A history of pneumonia, bronchitis, asthma, or other lung conditions
- Smoking
- Living or working in an area with high environmental pollution
- Neck, shoulder, and upper back problems
- Prolonged periods of stress or anxiety

Improving the Exchange Rate

Breathing low and slow tells your brain that everything is okay. When your brain thinks that you are in a state of high anxiety it shuts down the parasympathetic nervous system, taking blood away from body systems such as your digestion.

This means that you aren't able to absorb all the nutrients from your food properly. Even if you have the best diet in the world, if you're breathing in a way that activates your sympathetic nervous system you're never going to get the full benefit of the good foods that you choose to eat.

Abdominal breathing also improves the quality of air you body receives, as the best exchange of oxygen and CO_2 happens deep in the lungs. This has a positive impact on your physical health and your energy levels.

Additionally, breathing deeply gives your abdominal muscles the workout they need. Your muscles are designed to expand and contract, and when this doesn't happen the muscle doesn't develop properly. Breathing deeply can actually give you a flatter stomach.

So breathing properly reduces your stress levels, while also improving your digestion, nutrition, muscle tone, and energy.

Difficulty Letting Go

Many people experience 'email apnoea' or 'waking apnoea', where the breath is held during moments of stress. The slow rhythm of inhaling and exhaling is replaced by a sudden intake of breath, which is then held rather than released.

It's very easy, in a stressful work environment, to lose awareness of the natural rhythm of breathing. As a result, it is increasingly common for people to forget to release the breath for periods of time, leading to physical and mental exhaustion, and impacting on how people feel about their work environment and their colleagues.

It is important to feel driven and motivated in the workplace, in order to ensure we take action, and this does require a certain amount of tension. This is fine. After all, the sympathetic and parasympathetic nervous systems are designed to work together. However, living in a constant state of high anxiety is very unhealthy.

In The Workplace – Case Study
Margaret - Email Apnoea

Margaret was very aware of her wellbeing, and really conscious of being healthy. However, after observing Margaret in her workplace during a number of meetings, I noticed that she was holding her breath when she was working.

This is a phenomenon called 'email apnoea'. You may be familiar with the term 'sleep apnoea'. Email apnoea, or waking apnoea, is a similar thing, where you actually stop breathing.

Linda Stone, a former Apple executive, coined the term email apnoea. It occurs when you're in prolonged periods of concentration, and you hold your breath without realising.

As with sleep apnoea, it's significantly under-diagnosed. However, the breath work teacher, Dr. Belisa Vranich, states in her book, *Breathe,* that three out of ten people she meets in the workplace are breath holders. This makes email apnoea a significant phenomenon.

Email apnoea is something our modern lifestyle has created. Breath holding is something we would have done in the past when were in a state of heightened concentration while stalking an animal, to ensure that we did not alert it to our presence. It's not a technique that was designed to be used while sitting at a desk, typing away on a computer.

As a result of her breath holding, Margaret found that she was getting quite a lot of headaches. Throughout her meetings, Margaret would hold her breath, then all of a sudden she'd take a deep inhale, which sometimes caused her to snort. She was embarrassed by this, and really wanted to find a solution.

I suggested that she get a little piece of medical tape, and place it over her mouth. See the exercise 'Keep Your Mouth Shut' on page 47 for more information of how to use this technique.

I recommended that she keep the tape in place for an hour, while she was working. Taping your mouth gives you the awareness to continually breathe through your nose. This awareness teaches your body to notice whether you're holding your breath. Using a balanced breathing technique, breathing in through your nose and out through your nose, for a count of four, further enhances this awareness.

After using this technique for two or three weeks, Margaret realised that her headaches had gone, and people in the office were no longer asking if she was alright when she suddenly took a sharp inhale of breath. She also found that she was able to get a lot more work done, because she was able to concentrate for longer periods of time.

Conscious Breathing for Business

In the last twenty or thirty years there has been a huge explosion in breathwork, with practitioners exploring natural highs and altered states, as well as developing techniques to combat difficulties with health conditions such as sleep apnoea and asthma.

Contrary to some of the messages you may have received about modern breathwork practices, you don't need to plunge yourself into ice baths, sit cross-legged at the top of a snow-capped mountain, or retreat to a designated sacred space in order to practice conscious breathing. Equally, you don't need to hyperventilate or learn how to free dive to improve your breathing.

Breathing in a way that benefits how you navigate your working day only needs to involve simple, practical techniques. Conscious breathing does not need to be complex. Although some of the techniques may seem strange when you are first introduced to them, they very quickly become second nature.

Some of the practices in this book are things that you can learn at home, and then take into a work environment once you are comfortable and confident about what you are doing.

When you have mastered the techniques that we will be exploring, no one will be aware of the fact that you are practicing conscious breathing. The act of beneficial breathing is not obvious, although the effects are. By using a few quick, accessible tools you can change the way you operate in your daily life, in a professional and personal context.

Every aspect of the conscious breathing that we will be covering will make sense to you, with all the techniques and principles rooted in science. When you have a clear understanding of what is going on with your breathing, you can easily develop the awareness that enables you to know how to breathe in the ways that are most beneficial to your body and mind.

The outcomes you can achieve with beneficial breathing are improved concentration, lower stress levels, better communication, and a greater sense of wellbeing.

Key Takeaways

- Just because breathing happens naturally, this doesn't mean we shouldn't develop an awareness of how we are breathing. There is a difference between doing something, and doing it well.
- Conscious breathing can fast track you into being present, giving you the opportunity to take control and connect back into yourself.
- Beneficial breathing does not need to be complex, obvious, or time-consuming. You can make deep changes to your daily life with just a few simple conscious breathing techniques.
- Your body knows how to breathe well. The key is unlearning bad habits, so that you can put this intuitive knowledge into practice.

Are you wanting to connect with your breath and reduce stress?

Then contact Braith at: https://braithbamkin.com.au/#breathe_section to find out how he can help you personally.

Chapter Two

The Mechanics of Breathing

One of my teachers, Lucas Rockwood, constantly reminds us that the nose is for breathing and the mouth is for eating. Some of the exercises we are going to undertake in this book will require you to breathe through your mouth, as a practice of consciousness. However, the ultimate goal is to breathe through your nose whenever possible. When we breathe through our mouths we are not helping our respiratory system to function in the way it was designed to.

Before going into more detail about the mechanics of breathing, it is worth highlighting a couple of interesting points about the composition of air that you inhale and exhale, and the roles of oxygen and carbon dioxide.

The Air That You Breathe

The air that you inhale is composed of several different gases. Nitrogen accounts for a massive 79%, while oxygen is just 20.95% of the total. There are also small amounts of argon, neon, helium, and hydrogen, as well as carbon dioxide, which makes up just 0.04% of inhaled air.

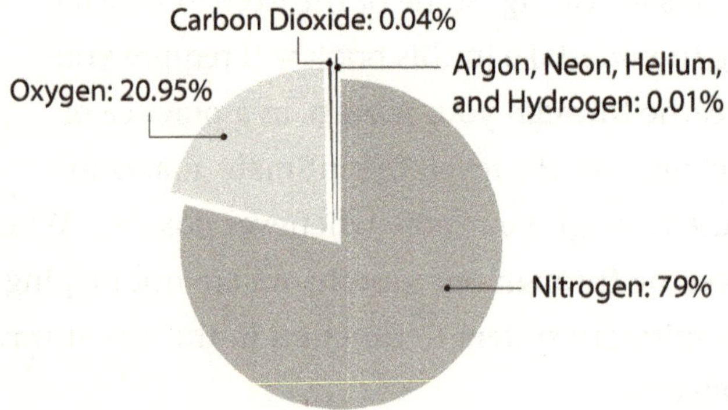

The air that you exhale contains a far greater amount of carbon dioxide – about 100 times as much, in fact, at around 4%. As you might expect, less oxygen is exhaled, accounting for roughly 15% of the total, while the nitrogen level remains the same, at 79%. Between 5% and 6% of the air you breathe out is water vapour, and the remainder is comprised of small amounts of argon, hydrogen, carbon monoxide, ammonia, and volatile organic compounds that your body wants to get rid of.

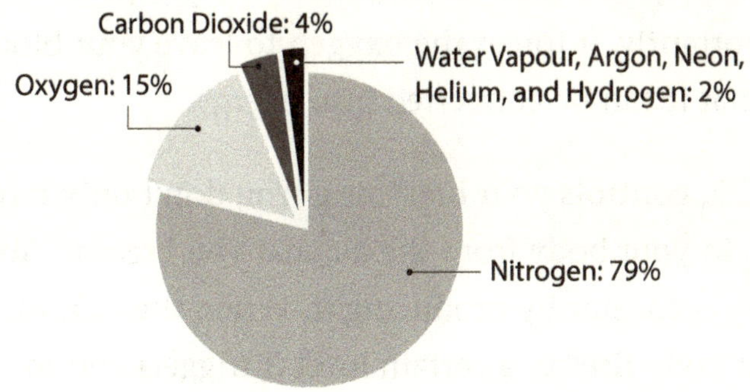

The Role of Oxygen

You need energy for your body to function. In order for your body to access this energy it combines sugar, sourced from the carbohydrates you eat, with oxygen, sourced from the air you breathe.

Digestion breaks carbohydrates down into sugars, which can then pass into your blood. The blood then carries the sugars to all the cells throughout your body. Once the sugars reach the cells, their chemical bond is broken and the energy is released. In order to break the chemical bond, your cells need oxygen.

The Role of Carbon Dioxide

Carbon dioxide, or CO_2, is often viewed as a waste product, but this is not quite true. CO_2 helps your body in a number of different ways. Most importantly, it forces the oxygen to leave your blood so that it can be converted into energy.

CO_2 controls your breathing. You don't only have CO_2 in your body from the air that you breathe. Your body is constantly producing it. When the CO_2 in your body rises to a certain level it triggers you to breathe in. When you breathe out, you expel the CO_2 from your body, and then the whole cycle begins again.

Although it seems counterintuitive, the more CO_2 you have in your system, the more oxygen you are able to absorb. This is why people are given a paper bag to breathe into when they are having a panic attack. The increased level of CO_2 that they take in from breathing into the bag increases the level of oxygen their bodies are able to uptake.

Understanding the composition of air and the way your body uses oxygen and carbon dioxide enables you to see that breathing is fundamental to your physical and mental wellbeing. The next step is to understand the mechanics of breathing, so that you can maximise the benefits.

The Nose

How you take the air into your body is the first step to maximising the benefits of breathing. This is why breathing through your nose is so important. There are several reasons for this, the first of which is that your nose is designed to filter out as much particulate matter as possible.

The nasal hairs, nasal mucosa, sinus passages, and sinuses are designed to catch all of the unwanted particles in the air. If you breathe through your mouth, there is no filtration system whatsoever. Mouth breathing means that everything in the air goes straight into your body.

When you breathe through your nose, the breath is taken through the sinus passages into the sinuses, which are cavities in your face and skull. There are four pairs of sinuses, collectively called the paranasal sinuses.

The sinuses produce nitric oxide, which has antimicrobial properties, providing a further line of defence against any impurities that have found their way through the sinus passages.

The Lungs

Nitric oxide also helps dilate the blood vessels, so that once the air reaches the lungs, they can absorb oxygen more efficiently. As less than 21% of the air that you breathe is oxygen, nitric oxide plays a very important role in helping your body uptake the oxygen.

Another advantage of breathing through the nose is that once the air reaches the sinus passages it is then taken in a very directed way into the lungs. On the other hand, when you breathe through your mouth the air is directed into the lungs in a very turbulent fashion. Think of breathing through your mouth as sending a 'fire hose' blast of air into your lungs, as opposed to breathing through your nose, which gives you a controlled and manageable volume of air, more of a 'garden hose' delivery method. This makes it more difficult for the air to reach all the alveoli, which are the tiny air sacs in your lungs that take up the oxygen and give back the CO_2.

The lungs are big – in fact if you stretched them out flat they would take up an area of around 80 to 100 square metres, or about half a tennis court. If you can imagine how folded up they must be to fit inside your chest, it becomes apparent that the air we breathe has quite a journey to go on in order to reach the point where our body can make the best use of it.

Imagine that your lungs are shaped somewhat like traffic cones, with the majority of the surface area located at the bottom of your lungs. In order to access that large area at the bottom of the 'traffic cone', it is important that we learn to breathe in an anatomically correct way.

How Breathing Is Measured

There are two different ways that the amount of air you breathe is measured - **lung volume** and **lung capacity**.

There are four units of lung volume, **tidal volume**, which is the amount of air you inhale and exhale in one normal breath, **inspiratory reserve volume**, which is how much more air you can breathe in after one normal inhale, **expiratory reserve volume**, which is how much more air you can breathe out after one normal exhale, and **residual volume,** which is the amount of air left in your lungs after you breathe out the expiratory reserve volume of your lungs. Residual volume exists because your lungs are never completely empty.

Lung capacity measures two or more lung volumes. Your **vital capacity** measures the maximum amount of air that you can inhale or exhale. It is calculated by adding together your tidal volume and both your inspiratory and expiratory reserve volumes. You can increase your vital capacity through exercise and conscious breathing.

Your **total lung capacity** is the total amount of air that your lungs can hold. It is calculated by adding together all four units of your lung volume. Most adults have a **total lung capacity** of between four and six litres, depending on a variety of factors including height, gender, and whether you grew up on a mountain or by the sea.

Your **breathing rate** is the number of breaths you take in a minute. The average breathing rate for an adult is twelve breaths a minute. The average tidal volume is 500 millilitres. **Minute ventilation** is how much air enters your lungs in one minute. The average minute ventilation is six litres a minute, which is equivalent to the upper limit of total lung capacity.

In The Workplace – Air Conditioning And Heating Systems

Air conditioning systems work by taking moisture out of the air. Of course this makes the air very dry. If you are breathing through your mouth you are constantly expelling huge amounts of water, and in an air-conditioned environment you can quickly become dehydrated.

Breathing through your nose not only prevents you from losing water, it also ensures the air that is reaching your lungs is at the correct temperature. Breathing in air that is below body temperature is not healthy, and will stress your system.

Additionally, office air conditioning units often don't have efficient filtration systems, which means that if your place of work relies on air conditioning to keep the space cool, the air you breathe is going to be full of the bugs that your co-workers are carrying.

Interestingly, aeroplanes have very efficient air conditioning systems. If you travel regularly for work you may have concerns about the air conditioning putting you at risk of catching other people's bugs. As aeroplanes have such good filtration systems, you are far more likely to get sick from air travel as a result of breathing cooler, drier air. Breathing through your nose can help to counteract this problem.

Heating systems can also be extremely problematic, as the warmer air can encourage viruses to grow. In a shared office environment, this is another reason why breathing through your nose is far more beneficial.

During Covid-19 it was shown that patients in single rooms in hospitals in were expelling the virus, which was then getting into the ventilation systems and being carried throughout the hospital. As a result, hospitals have been doing a lot of work on improving their air filtration systems. This is another clear demonstration of why it is important to breathe correctly.

Causes and Effects of Mouth Breathing

Breathing through the mouth may happen for a variety of reasons, including nasal congestion, enlarged tonsils, a deviated septum, the shape of your nose or jaw, problems with allergies and asthma, as well as stress and anxiety.

Mouth breathing often results from existing problems, and it may also cause a variety of new problems, such as bad breath and poor oral health, decreased lung function, and lower levels of oxygen in the blood, – which is associated with heart failure and high blood pressure.

The Advantages of Breathing Efficiently

The slang term 'mouth breather' is an insult for the very reason that we instinctively know there is something wrong and unhealthy about breathing through the mouth rather than the nose.

High performance athletes are taught to breathe through the nose, because they get much better results when they do so. The temptation to breathe through the mouth may be strong, but when we learn to use our breath in a controlled manner, we are able to maximise the way in which we are designed to breathe.

You may have observed from watching the Olympics or similar sporting competitions, that after people do the 100-metre sprint, they lean forward, place their hands on their knees, and breathe deeply through their mouths. This is called the 'tripod position', and it allows the diaphragm to work more efficiently. In this situation, where you need to get as much air as possible into your lungs, breathing through the mouth is preferable. This is because the mouth is bigger than the nose, and so you can intake a higher volume of air much more quickly.

When you are breathing efficiently and taking the air deep into your lungs where the best oxygen and CO_2 exchange takes place, all your body systems are able to function smoothly. As discussed in Chapter One, this means that your digestion is more efficient, your energy levels are higher, and your concentration is improved. Even your eyesight is affected.

When you are stressed and your sympathetic nervous system is engaged, your pupils dilate so that you are able to see further. In a relaxed state you do not need to see long distances. This makes it easier to concentrate on looking at things close up, such as your computer screen, and you are less likely to experience headaches caused by eyestrain and bright lighting.

Example –Breathing For Better Health

I was born with a deviated septum and had severe asthma throughout my childhood. As a result, I breathed through my mouth a lot of the time.

In spite of the fact that I was super fit and ate

really well, the mouth breathing caused me all sorts of problems, such as frequent sore throats, ulcers, and colds.

I also had problems with snoring and sleep apnoea. I would never wake up feeling refreshed, and was constantly tired throughout the day.

Following a sleep study, when it was confirmed that I had sleep apnoea, I started to use a constant positive airways pressure machine, referred to as a CPAP. CPAPs help you to breathe consistently through the night, by directing a steady stream of airflow, which ramps up automatically if you have a case of apnoea. As I could only wear the device over my nose, I was forced to breath through my nose.

Within weeks, I stopped having sore throats, I stopped getting ulcers, I stopped catching every cold going around, I had more energy, and I could easily get through the day without feeling exhausted.

The reason that all these changes took place so rapidly is that the nose is designed for breathing, and I was now breathing, anatomically and biomechanically, in the way I was designed to. The results in my life were spectacular.

Exercise – Keep Your Mouth Shut

If you are a chronic mouth breather, or used to breathing through your mouth during exercise, then making the switch to breathing through your nose can feel confronting.

Take a walk around your neighbourhood, so that the exercise is not too vigorous, with a small piece of surgical tape over your mouth. This will force you to breathe through your nose. As surgical tape can be easily removed it will not prevent you from breathing through your mouth in the event of an emergency, as it will just pop off if you take a big breath in through your mouth.

If you have sensitive skin it is advisable to apply a little lip balm before placing the tape across your mouth. For everyone, it's wise to roll your lips slightly inwards so that the tape isn't on the sensitive part of your lips (although this may be difficult is you have facial hair). The idea is to use a small piece of tape placed vertically across the centre of your mouth, rather than a long strip along the full length of your mouth. Think of the size of the piece of tape as a small postage stamp.

By practicing moving at a reasonable pace with your mouth taped closed you should quickly find that you are able to take part in more vigorous exercise without your mouth taped up, and still continue to breathe through your nose.

This method can also be used if you are inclined to breathe through your mouth while you sleep. Good indications that you are breathing through your mouth when you are asleep are if you wake up with a very dry throat, and that you feel very thirsty.

Taping your mouth at night will have the same effect as during exercise. Again, if you need to take a big gasp of breath it will not stop you, as the tape will simply come off.

When you want to take the tape off, if you purse your lips inwards then you can easily remove the tape without irritating the sensitive skin of your mouth.

Posture

From a very young age we are taught to sit up straight when we need to pay attention. This is because we know that when our body is in an upright position, we are most able to engage with the environment around us.

When we slump, it is a false sense of relaxation. We are not able to expand our abdomen properly, which means we cannot get enough air into our lungs, and our brain receives the message that we are in a state of anxiety.

The best way to breathe is to sit up straight, relax your shoulders, and to breathe deeply from your abdomen. We are designed to sit up straight, with relaxed shoulders, and to breathe deeply into our abdomen, expanding horizontally, low and slow. When you look at people who breathe really well, such as singers and those who meditate, you may notice that their postures seem correct. It is very easy for us to intuitively see what good posture looks like.

If you are asked to sit or stand in a comfortable position that you need to hold for a long time, you will tend to naturally adopt a posture that is helpful to your breathing. You instinctively know what to do. However, it is easy to sink into bad postural habits caused by inappropriate furniture and physical tension. Correcting your posture is often a question of remembering something you already know.

In The Workplace – Furniture And Screens

Our modern lifestyles, from the sofas we relax on at home, to the desks we sit behind at work, have had an adverse effect on our posture. All too often, particularly at work, we bend forward.

Standing desks, computers at eye-height, ergonomic chairs, fit balls, and a variety of other options have been gaining popularity in recent years, and all of these options can greatly assist your posture. However, the simple truth is that we were not designed to sit for eight hours at a time staring at a screen.

You have probably heard that we are meant to take a screen break every twenty minutes, and get up and walk around every half an hour, but for many people this simply isn't possible. This is why ensuring you have the correct posture and breathing technique is vital.

Costal Breathing and Diaphragmatic Breathing

Costal breathing, or shallow breathing, engages the intercostal muscles, which are the muscles that run between the ribs. These muscles contract when you inhale, and relax as you exhale. If you are breathing from high in your chest then you are often only using your intercostal and accessory muscles.

Costal breathing causes a great deal of tension in your shoulders, and does not draw the air deep into your lungs. You are likely to get tired much more quickly when you are breathing in this way.

Diaphragmatic breathing, abdominal breathing, and deep breathing are all the same thing. The thoracic diaphragm, often simply called the diaphragm, is a large, curved sheet of muscle that separates the chest cavity from the abdomen.

When you inhale, your diaphragm engages and moves downwards, making more space in your chest cavity for your lungs to expand. When you exhale, your diaphragm relaxes and moves upwards. A good way to picture how your diaphragm works is to think of it as being like a jellyfish, flattening with the in-breath and curving with the out-breath. Like a jellyfish, the diaphragm is circular, and runs around the middle of your entire torso.

Diaphragmatic breathing is relaxing, and creates the space in your body for you to breathe efficiently. This way of breathing reduces physical and mental tension, and sustains your energy levels. It also helps to carry the air to the alveoli. As the alveoli are the last stop on the line in the network of your lungs, breathing deeply is really important in ensuring the best possible oxygen and CO_2 exchange takes place.

Not only this, but breathing is responsible for eliminating up to 70% of all waste products from your body – not just the toxins you breathe, but the toxins you ingest through eating and drinking. Breathing deeply helps you to get rid of these toxins more effectively and efficiently.

The Vagus Nerve

Understanding your vagus nerve and the function it plays is essential to understanding correct breathing. The word 'vagus' shares its etymology with the word 'vagabond', both coming from the Latin 'to wander', which is a good description of how the vagus nerve functions.

The vagus nerve stretches out from the base of your brain into many of your major organs, creating pathways to your heart, lungs, digestive tract, diaphragm, and abdomen.

These vagal pathways govern your autonomic nervous system, creating calm or alarm, and leading to involuntary physical responses including increased heart rate, butterflies in your tummy, or relaxed breathing, depending on the circumstances.

When you sense danger, your vagal operations become restricted, triggering the stress response that prepares you for fight or flight. If the danger is extreme, your vagal operations shut down, causing you to freeze.

Diaphragmatic breathing stimulates and massages the vagus nerve, activating the vagal pathways. This slows your heart rate, relaxes the body, and improves decision-making, counteracting the fight, flight, or freeze response.

The Whole Is Greater Than The Sum Of Its Parts

Every stage of the mechanics of breathing works together as part of a carefully designed system that maximises your wellbeing, helping you to achieve and maintain the physical health and mental clarity that are the foundations of success and fulfilment in your professional and personal life.

Key Takeaways

- The nose is for breathing and the mouth is for eating!
- The air that we breathe isn't all oxygen. Carbon dioxide plays a significant role.
- Sitting up straight, with your shoulders relaxed, and breathing deeply from your abdomen enables you to get the greatest benefit from the air that you breathe.
- Your diaphragm is like a jellyfish in the centre of your body.

Chapter Three

Fasten Your Own Oxygen Mask First

When I was young adult, new technology was being delivered. The expectation was that it was going to reduce our workload. However, over the last thirty years of my working life, rather than helping us to reduce our workload, we've become a slave to technology, and our workload has actually increased.

Technology gives us access to information, people, places, and experiences that would have been unimaginable just a few years ago. Although there are great advantages to this unprecedented level of access, it is not purely a force for good. Many people feel very disconnected in their lives, work, and world.

One of the primary reasons for this is that humanity has a negativity bias. This was useful to us in the development of our species, because having a heightened awareness of things that may have harmed us kept us safe. These days, our negativity bias is evidenced by the way the media feeds us a constant stream of 'bad' news, as these are the stories that grab our attention.

However, receiving a never-ending flow of bad news can quickly lead to feelings of stress, anxiety, overwhelm, and powerlessness.

The advent of social media has created yet another platform that pulls us towards our negativity bias. Make no mistake, the owners of social media platforms have teams of people ensuring you engage with their site. Platforms are designed to be addictive, in order to have you come back over and over again. Unchecked, engaging with social media has us drawing endless comparisons with other people's lives in a way that creates feelings of dissatisfaction and inadequacy. As a result of this, a lot of energetic negativity is generated.

Many of us use social media in the workplace, and we can easily be drawn down the rabbit hole of negativity. The internet has changed the workplace forever, and the speed of that change is only going to increase.

One recent example of this is the Covid-19 crisis. From the outset, traditional news media and social media constantly fed us stories. I quickly made a conscious decision to curate my own news sources, and consumed the minimal amount required to understand what I needed in order to function in society. I observed that friends and colleagues of mine who were immersed in news and social platforms were becoming increasingly agitated, and I heard even the most rational people say things that were completely irrational and fear-based.

It is clear to see that technology has enormous power to help us, while also having the power to be very detrimental to our wellbeing. As a result, it is crucial that we control our use of technology, rather than having our use of technology control us.

Turn Off And Tune In

There is now an expectation that you are switched on and plugged in 24/7. This is having a dramatic impact on people's lives. The delineation between work and personal time has been blurred, and Covid-19 has exacerbated this. We've proven that we can work from home, but many of us now work significantly more hours than we did when we went into the office, and our commute time has become part of the working day.

When it comes to our working lives, many of us cannot say 'no' or set healthy boundaries. This means that many people are now permanently contactable, with the expectation of an immediate response. Being self-aware enables you to say 'no'. Although your instinct may be to say 'yes' to everything, in order to grow your business or secure your promotion and continue climbing to where you want to be, saying 'no' is an extremely powerful tool.

As a business owner, I know that it is very tempting to take on everything that comes my way, and to be in endless meetings, even when they don't provide much benefit. Yet I have learned the power of being present, and saying 'no' has really changed the way I work. I have also observed this in others.

Saying 'no' can induce feelings of guilt and increase the low levels of anxiety that result from the lack of connection we have with ourselves, creating a snowball effect. However, the reality is that most things that happen at work are not a matter of life or death. The exception to this is the emergency professions, but these people more than anyone need to be fully present in order to be able to make the best decisions.

We've all been on a plane before, and so we all know about fastening your own oxygen mask first. There's a reason that airlines give this advice. You can't help and support other people until you have taken care of yourself. To live in a sustainable and healthy way, you need to look after yourself before looking after others. And conscious breathing gives you the break that you need to look after yourself.

24/7 connectivity may feel necessary, but it is not the most productive way of operating. You need to look after yourself in order to be able to take care of your teams, your colleagues, and your clients. If you haven't got your own oxygen mask in place, you cannot help the people around you.

Perspective Through Presence

Being stressed makes it difficult to see things from other people's point of view. When people around you are reacting in crazy or unhelpful ways, unless you are fully present you can react to the craziness, and that's never a good thing. It's important to remember that you don't always know what's going on in someone else's life. It's not your job to fix other people's problems, but you can take responsibility for the way you respond to other people, and the way in which you engage with external stressors. By taking responsibility, you gain a lot more clarity around the questions you need to ask and the boundaries you need to set. By being present to a situation, you can see things for what they are.

Gaining this perspective allows you stop taking on other people's problems, which means that you can say 'no' to people. More than this, it means that the way in which you say no is measured, calm, rational, and reasonable. When you approach situations with this mindset, the way in which the other person is able to hear and receive your 'no' is much more likely to be understanding and accepting.

Everything on the planet is energy.

Neurons release chemicals, known as neurotransmitters. These neurotransmitters generate electrical signals in other neurons. The electrical signals then get transmitted to more and more neurons, which creates a thought.

This means that every thought is formed by a spark of electrical energy. You can sense that energy. When you walk into a room, you can often tell when someone's in a good mood or a bad mood. You can feel 'good vibes' from people, and sense when you're around people who are feeling happy or feeling negative. This is the energy that people are putting into the world.

When you are present, relaxed, and calm this is reflected in your thought processes, and so what you put out into the world adds to the sum total of positive energy. When you are anxious, stressed, and tense, the opposite is true. In both cases, people react accordingly, because energy is transmitted and received.

Think of it this way - when you turn your radio on, sound comes out. You can't see the radio waves, but you know they are there, carrying the sound. Equally, when you flick a light switch on, you know that electricity is illuminating the bulb. You can see the light, but you can't see the electricity.

Human beings are exactly the same. We give and receive energy through our thoughts, which in turn inform our behaviours. On a physical level, the brain, in combination with the spinal cord, comprises the central nervous system.

For this reason, it is really important to be very aware of having good posture and keeping your spinal cord straight and erect.

In Indian tradition, there are seven chakras, or energy centres, located along the length of the spine and up into the head. These chakras comprise the root chakra, located at the base of the spine, the sacral chakra, located just below the belly button, the solar plexus chakra, located in the upper abdomen, the heart chakra, located in the centre of the chest, the throat chakra, located in the neck, the brow chakra, located on the forehead, the crown chakra,

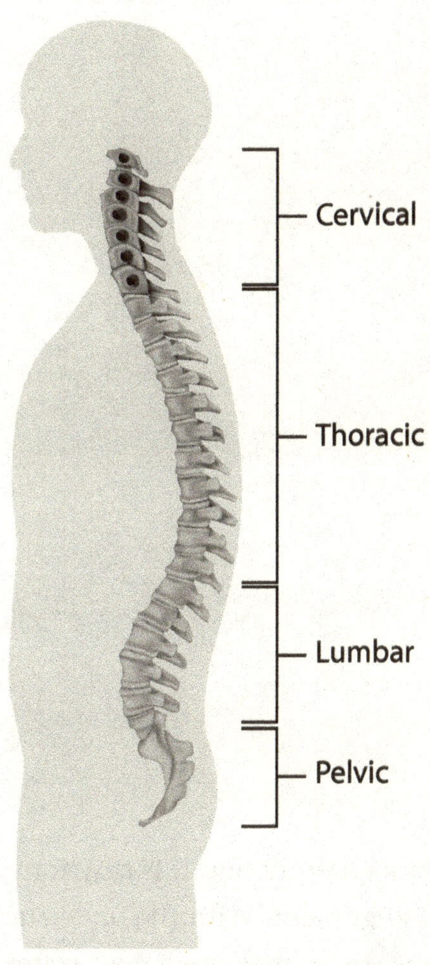

located on the very top of the head. There is also an eighth chakra, external to the body. This is often referred to as the star chakra, and is located a few inches above your head.

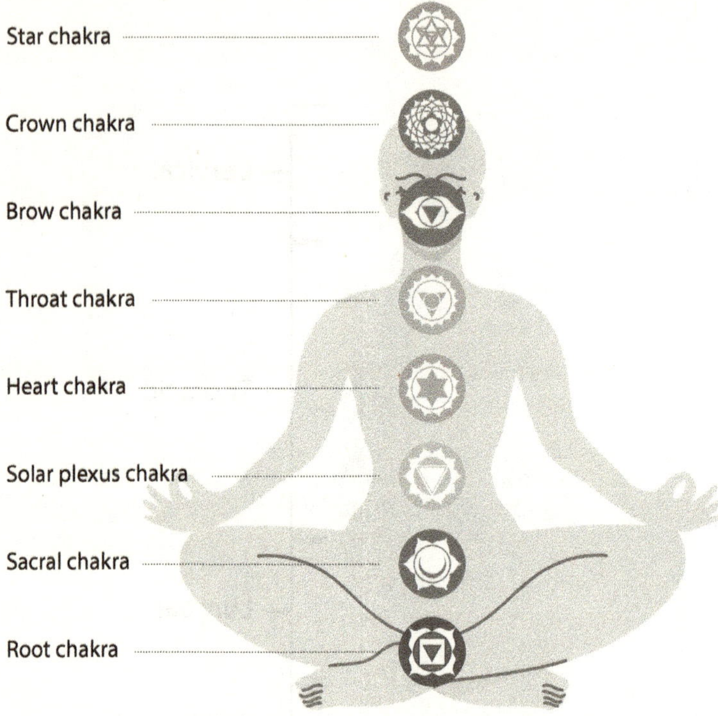

In a work environment it is easy for your spine to get out of alignment. With the understanding that the chakras are located along your spine, so that your spine transmits energy, if your spine is out of alignment then you're blocking the smooth flow of that energy.

One of the ways you can bring yourself into alignment on a psychological level, so that you are putting out positive thoughts and giving off positive energy, is to be connected to yourself. And one of the fastest ways of connect to yourself is through conscious breathing.

In The Workplace - Example
Breathe Through It

Recently, I had a situation where I had a disagreement with a supplier in my business about the way things were working. We had a meeting to negotiate the way in which we were going to move forward. I had created a lot of anxiety about the situation, and so when I arrived at the meeting, my supplier could sense the tension. As a result, the meeting was not going well, so I excused myself, went to the bathroom, shut myself in the cubicle, and sat down with my hands on my knees. I put my spine upright and did some simple four by four balancing breathing.

I could feel the energy moving calmly up and down my body, I could feel my heart and my brain in alignment, and I brought myself out of my head, into my body, and back into the present. This only took a couple of minutes.

Once I felt calm, I went back to the meeting, and the way we interacted completely changed. First of all, I felt better, so I was clear about what I needed to say. Secondly, he could sense a positive shift in my energy, so his reaction to me was completely different.

The second half of the meeting moved in a really different way. Even though I have a very good awareness of my energy, my anxiety had caused me to stop putting my attention into connecting to myself. Once I realised what was happening and changed it, the experience was much more positive for both of us.

We still didn't agree on an outcome and ended up parting ways, but we parted ways on a good note. The meeting finished, we shook hands, and we may well work together at a future stage, because that bridge hasn't been burned.

You don't have to believe in chakras and Eastern spirituality to know that energy can get stuck in your body. You can feel it intuitively.

Negative Energy Release Exercise

Heart Energy

Sit up straight in a chair, with your feet flat on the floor and your spine erect and slightly away from the back of your chair.

Without changing the pattern of your breathing, take a breath out and a breath in, then slowly breathe in for four breaths, then out for four breaths.

Concentrate on your breath coming in and out of your heart. Even though it's moving through your belly, feel it coming through your heart, moving slowly in and out through your heart. As you're doing that, generate a feeling of love, positivity, happiness and joy. The way in which you do that is to think of someone you love, a place that is your happy place, or an uplifting experience that's happened recently.

As you're breathing in and out through your heart, feel that energy in your heart. As you're doing this, your heart is sending this message to your brain. Although you may intuitively think that your brain is sending information to your heart, in fact, your heart has many more neurons than your brain and so the opposite is true.

Breathe these positive energy feelings for just two or three minutes, with your eyes open or closed, breathing slowly and calmly, and generating that sensation with your heart. In this way, you'll be telling your brain to change your state. This change can happen really quickly.

This exercise is something you can do throughout the day, and people don't even need to be aware that you're doing it.

Once you have completed the exercise, just come back to your normal routine and you'll notice a shift has taken place.

Negative Energy Release Exercise

Smiling Energy

Your body can't tell the difference between fake happiness and real happiness, which is where the power lies in this exercise.

Sit up straight in a chair, with your feet flat on the floor and your spine erect and slightly away from the back of your chair, breathing in deeply, through your abdomen.

As you're doing this, smile. Smile with your eyes, and smile with your mouth as you're breathing in and out through your nose. You don't have to smile widely. Just the gentle sensation of smiling is enough. All you need is to be able to feel it internally. The sensation of you smiling will tell your brain that everything's okay and that you're happy.

Continue to smile while breathing, slowly and softly, deeply into your abdomen, in and out, for a count of four. This tells your brain that everything's okay and that you're happy.

> You can do it with your eyes open or closed, just simply sit there and smile. Think about something that makes you happy. Sometimes it can be hard to smile, so if you're finding it hard to smile with your eyes, or to create a genuine smile of happiness or contentment, just raise the corners of your mouth. Even this can have a massive shift in the way you feel. When you combine this with a simple four-four breathing exercise, it's very powerful.

Moving your energy takes commitment, practice, and effort. You need to consciously work to get the result that you're looking for. Uncomfortable feelings naturally arise when you are confronted by something that is uncomfortable. It's what you then do about those feelings, and how you bring yourself into a state of being that creates a positive energy that is key to creating a positive outcome.

Tip On The Tightrope

Our body is not in stasis. We are constantly making incremental shifts that affect our physical and emotional balance. Like a tightrope walker, we perform minute corrections that keep the momentum moving forward, continuously adjusting between the two states of sympathetic and parasympathetic nervous systems – fight/flight and rest/digest.

Although people put value judgements on these two states, neither of them is good or bad. It's really important to understand that we need both the sympathetic and parasympathetic nervous systems. For instance, we need the sympathetic nervous system to compel us to take action.

In a work context, without the sympathetic nervous system we would never have the impetus to meet deadlines, the courage to give presentations, or the drive to scale. All of these things are hugely beneficial to our professional lives, and so in this context stress is not bad. However, it needs to be countered with the parasympathetic nervous system so that we can come to rest, rather than constantly being in a state of movement. We need to attain and maintain a healthy balance. As with everything in life, too much of a good thing can easily become a bad thing.

Striking The Balance

Your nervous system moves between sympathetic and parasympathetic every hour and a half to three hours, naturally cycling between these two different states of being. You may recognise this from the understanding that it is extremely difficult to sit in place and focus on a task for four hours.

The reason it is so difficult to sit in place for this length of time is that your nervous system is going to switch from sympathetic and parasympathetic at least once during a four-hour period. As a result, a couple of hours into a work task you may get up and madly vacuum the house. Alternatively, after a couple of hours of focused work you might find that you are very sleepy and your thoughts escape you. This is completely normal.

The cycle of your sympathetic and parasympathetic nervous systems is aligned to your breathing. Throughout the day, your breathing switches from being left-nostril dominant to being right-nostril dominant. This is the case for approximately ninety per cent of people.

When the parasympathetic nervous system is engaged, the left nostril is dominant, and vice versa. The sympathetic nervous system is very task-orientated, and so understanding and working with this natural cycle of dominant nostril breathing can really help performance levels and targets.

You can test which nostril is dominant by putting your finger under your nose when you breathe. It is a great indication of where you are at, and can be applied in many different situations.

For example, if you go to the gym and find that you are struggling with your workout, by putting your finger under your nose you may be able to determine from your breathing that you are at a point in your cycle where your parasympathetic nervous system is engaged. If this is the case, your body will want to rest, rather than engage in activity.

Slave To The Rhythm?

The brilliant news is that you do not need to be a slave to this cycle. With a few simple breathing exercises you can change whether your sympathetic or parasympathetic nervous system is engaged.

Most people don't understand how to make the shift between one state and the other, and so there is an acceptance that it is simply the way they are feeling at that point in time. However, it is very easy to change from the sympathetic to the parasympathetic system, and vice versa. The exercises that enable this are covered in later chapters.

As it is completely normal to go between the two states over the course of the day, these shifts in our cycle are something that are simply a part of how we operate. Neither state is good or bad – they are both natural and needed. Even so, changing the cycle is completely fine.

The reason why it is fine to change the cycle is that the body is designed to react to external stimuli. Going all the way back through our history as a species, being able to instantly react to danger has been paramount to our survival. You need to be able to take action and get moving. So being able to engage the sympathetic nervous system in a split second is essential. Equally, once the danger has passed, you don't want to remain in a state of anxiety.

Examples – Sympathetic And Parasympathetic Switch

We're designed to respond to our external environment in a way that is appropriate. You can see this in action when you watch sprinters cross the finish line. The first thing they do is put their hands on their thighs and gasp for air. They engaged their sympathetic nervous system and pushed all the oxygen into their heart, lungs, and muscles to carry themselves through the race. Once the race is over, they need to bring in as much air as possible to rebalance their system. They need to be able to switch back to the parasympathetic nervous system taking the dominant role.

Another good example of switching between states is during physical intimacy. In order to achieve arousal, you need to be able to relax. In a state of high anxiety, arousal isn't possible, and so your parasympathetic nervous system needs to be engaged. At the point of release, however, the sympathetic nervous system engages.

These are examples of your body governing the switch. But making that change between sympathetic and parasympathetic is something you can consciously take control over. Feelings of anxiety can be greatly reduced by understanding how to engage the parasympathetic nervous system and bring yourself into a state of calm.

Unhealthy Addictions

Many people are very quick to turn to legal and illegal drugs, alcohol, cigarettes, and food in an attempt to change their state of being. It is possible to become very reliant on these things in order to feel in control.

This need to take control of your state of being is absolutely understandable. However, rather than looking outside yourself for the solutions, you can very easily achieve the changes you want to bring about through your breathing.

There are habits that are going to support you in really productive ways, and those that are very detrimental to your wellbeing. Modern life, particularly in Western societies, is structured in a way that bombards you with information, giving you massive releases of dopamine and cortisol, which spin you from dramatic highs to crashing lows.

Companies want you to become addicted to their products. Subliminal and overt messages about how much better your life would be if you had the bright and shiny things are all-pervasive, and the rise of social media has greatly increased marketing opportunities. Social media is not designed to connect us to one another. It is designed to sell to us. These platforms are massive vehicles for advertising.

It is so important to remember this. The ways in which we are encouraged to connect with one another, both for business and in our personal lives, can be a source of great anxiety for many people. If we are not fully present and aware of what is going on around us then the world will happen to us. When this is the case, of course we feel overwhelmed and out of control.

Craving engagement is natural, but understanding the aims of social media enables us to make choices about how we engage. Do these things use us, or do we use them? Used properly, social media can be a great tool for staying connected.

Defining when, where, and how you make use of online resources is central to maintaining balance and control. Stepping away from other people's narratives is essential. The tension that arises when we get drawn in can be very damaging. If you find yourself becoming anxious when using social media, taking a break and practicing some simple deep breathing techniques will help you to rebalance yourself.

When you're really present you can make healthy choices. Conscious breathing is a very important component of taking control and choosing how you react. It is very empowering to know you have a choice about whether to go with the monkey-mind chatter and to buy into the idea that you are inadequate, or to let go of that way of thinking.

When we start to believe that we are not ok, or that we need to compare ourselves to others, that's when we start to detach from ourselves. Being able to breathe into your body brings you back to your true nature, and the realisation that your true nature is good.

A conscious choice that I made in my late teens, after a period of depression and suicidal ideation, was that being happy was easier than being unhappy. It takes a lot more energy to be unhappy than to be happy, but so many people become addicted to the negativity bias that it can be very hard to see this truth clearly.

What I love about conscious breathing is that, even if it's just for a couple of minutes, it pulls you away from the negative mental chatter. When you are focused on your breathing, the monkey mind becomes quiet and you can't concentrate on the fact that your client didn't like your proposal, or that your boss criticised your presentation, or that someone else got the promotion you had your heart set on. Just try it for yourself.

Exercise –
Letting Go of Negative Mental Chatter

Inhale for a count of four and exhale for a count of four. Really focus on the breath, and the sensations in your body as you inhale and exhale. Continue this pattern of breathing in and out for a count of four for two minutes.

Unless you are breathing in a way that supports your nervous system, having a positive mindset is going to be hugely challenging. In order to have a positive mindset, you need to be able to manage your nervous system in a constructive way. This means consciously moving between sympathetic and parasympathetic, and knowing when you need to change from one to the other, or having your body naturally move between these two states in an appropriate way.

There are times where you need to take action, and times when you need to be in a state of calm. Understanding which state you need to be in, and how to use your breathing to achieve each state, is central to your wellbeing.

Key Takeaways

- Looking after yourself is key to a balanced life.
- Being in control of good posture helps with your energy.
- Shifting between the sympathetic and parasympathetic nervous systems is natural and needed.
- Using conscious breathing to become fully present reduces anxiety and creates clarity, enabling you to make better decisions and set healthy boundaries.

Chapter Four

Energising, Balancing, And Calming Breathing

Energy is the new commodity, and breath fuels this valuable resource. In this chapter, we will look at three breathing styles that you can harness to empower your life. I refer to these as energising, balancing, and calming.

You may have heard other practitioners talking about coffee, water, and whisky breathing, or uplifting and contemplative breathing. There are many other terms, including Sanskrit words, but no matter what the words used they all refer to breathing that is energising, balancing, and calming. These terms don't refer specifically to practices, but rather to a group of exercises that achieve the requisite result.

- Energising breathing enlivens you, and is best practised in the morning or when you need a pick-me-up during the day (however, refrain from using energising breathing in the evening).

- Balancing breathing stabilises you, and can be used at any time of the day or night.
- Calming breathing relaxes you, and is best used at the end of your working day, or around particularly stressful situations.

There isn't one of these three types of breathing that is better than the other two. There can often be a misconception that the focus always needs to be on calming breathing. The thinking is that it is beneficial to live in a state of perpetual relaxation. In reality, you need different levels of awareness and alertness at different points in time.

How Conscious Breathing Works

In Chapter Two we covered the mechanics of breathing. As we know, conscious breathing can change your blood pressure, your breathing rate, and your heart rate variability (HRV). Through these changes, you are able to adjust the levels of CO_2 and oxygen in your body.

Unless you are doing extreme versions of breathing, you won't dramatically change the levels of CO_2 and oxygen in your blood. None of the exercises in this book are extreme, and so the changes that occur in the CO_2 and oxygen levels in your blood will be slight, but the impact can still be significant. In the context of conscious breathing for the workplace slight changes are all that is needed.

With all the breathing exercises in this book, it is important to breathe through your nose whenever possible. But, if there is a reason why you cannot breathe through your nose, then there is no need to beat yourself up about it.

Sinus trouble, colds, allergies, and air conditioning can all affect nasal breathing. If this is the case, you can adapt the breathing exercises to mouth breathing, and still ensure you benefit from the effects. In general, as has been previously discussed, try to remember that the mouth is for eating and the nose is for breathing.

Equally, it is possible to relieve a blocked nose. The following exercises are very beneficial in helping to achieve this.

Exercise - Thirty Second Breath Hold

A lot of people suffer from blocked noses. You get sniffy and stuffy, with sinus problems caused by allergies or environmental pollutants. This can be quite debilitating, and in the workplace the problem can be exacerbated by air-conditioning systems and limited opportunities to go outside into the fresh air, leading to associated problems with headaches and eyestrain, which make it difficult to concentrate.

The good news is that there's a really easy way of relieving a blocked nose. Start by taking a deep breath in, low and slow, into your abdomen. This will probably need to be done through the mouth, if your nose is blocked. Inhale for a count of four and exhale for a count of four for two cycles. On the third cycle, inhale and gently hold your breath. It's important not to add any pressure to your rib cage, your facial cavity, or your cranial cavity by forcing yourself to hold your breath really hard. It's a light hold.

Ideally, you want to hold the breath for thirty

seconds. Close your eyes and count internally. If you can't make it to thirty seconds that's absolutely fine. As soon as you get breath hunger, breathe out. Once you have completed the third breath, start the pattern again, breathing in and out for two cycles of a count of four on the inhale and a count of four on the exhale. Then on the third cycle, hold your breath again for another thirty seconds, or as long as you can comfortably manage.

This exercise increases the CO_2 in your lungs and opens the nasal cavity. Repeat this exercise as often as you need to.

Exercise - Humming

This exercise is fun, and really calming. I like to use it on a regular basis and it is one of my favourite practices. A lot of cultures have a tradition of humming – and those of you who have been exposed to sound therapy may have come across this as well. It is also something that children naturally do to self-soothe, but as adults we have had these types of fun practices taken away from us.

Gently press your thumbs onto your tragus (the external triangular part of your ear that can block the ear canal if pressed inwards). Take a deep breath in for a count of four, and then hum as you slowly exhale from low in your abdomen for as long as you possibly can. The goal is to completely empty your lungs. There is no need to count the exhale. Repeat this for a couple of minutes.

It might seem a bit wacky if you're doing this in the office. So you may prefer to do it when there's nobody around, or in a quiet meeting room. In any case, your work colleagues will be intrigued by what you're doing, and will probably want to join in at some point.

This exercise is really beneficial in a couple of different ways. Firstly, it's super relaxing. This is because humming massages and stimulates the vagus nerve. Children naturally put their fingers in their ears and hum to calm themselves down, as it brings their external stimulation down.

The other reason that humming is beneficial is it stimulates nitric oxide in the nasal cavity, which helps dilate the blood vessels. Humming slowly to exhale completely, interspersed with regular inhales, is considered to be a calming breathing exercise.

Once again, you're building up the CO_2 in your lung capacity. So you've got the nitric oxide in your nasal cavity and the CO_2 in your lungs. This, in combination with the massaging of the vagus nerve, is extremely calming. So if you're feeling very worked up, this is a simple, quick fix to relax. Because it also helps to relieve your nasal blockage, this is considered a 'two for one' exercise.

Clothing

As we have seen previously, tight clothing can have a negative impact on your physiology. While you are learning to use conscious breathing in the comfort of your own home, make sure you are wearing loose fitting clothing, so that nothing restricts the flow of your breath.

If you are wearing tight and restrictive clothing to the workplace, you may be creating a situation where you're telling your body that you are stressed. Check and see how tight your clothing is, particularly around your waist and chest. If you can't breathe fully into your abdomen in a circular fashion, and your ribcage can't expand naturally to complement this, it is time to look honestly at your wardrobe.

Your fashion choices shouldn't be a contributor to your stress levels. When I share this information with clients, it is often a difficult conversation to have, but I have seen many people achieve instant results from releasing themselves from their restrictive garments. I invite you to be honest about how restricting your clothing is, and to enjoy the freedom that breathing fully and naturally can provide.

Energising Breathing

Energising breathing increases your breathing rate, raising the levels of oxygen and reducing the levels of carbon dioxide in your blood. This reduction in CO_2 is sometimes known as 'off-gassing'.

Energising breathing uses short, sharp exhales, pushing the air out of your lungs. It's a great practice to use when you are feeling flat. It can be a great technique for those points in the working day when you have hit a slump. Rather than reaching for a sugary snack or a caffeinated drink, you can reinvigorate yourself by carrying out an energising breathing exercise. You can also use it to prepare yourself for presentations, public speaking, a Zoom marathon, or a mid-afternoon meeting that you know will be mind-numbing.

Energising breathing is probably not a technique you want to practice in an open office. It is best done behind closed doors where you can be undisturbed for a few minutes, whether that is in your a private office, a break-out room, or another area in the workplace.

Energising breathing is a less extreme version of holotropic breathing, which can produce a natural high or altered state as a result of the reduction in CO_2. Holotropic breathing is essentially hyperventilation.

The exercises in this book do not cause extreme off-gassing and will not dramatically reduce the carbon dioxide levels in your blood. Even so, energising breathing still needs to be carried out with care and awareness. If you do start to feel light-headed when you are doing an energising breathing exercise, stop and take a breather. Literally.

Energising Exercise – Lion's Breath

If you've ever been to a yoga class, you may have done this Lion's Breath exercise.

Breathing in through your nose and then out through your mouth, really hard, with your tongue sticking out, so that you're making yourself look like a lion.

Breathe in through your nose for a count of four, and then push the air up from below your navel, and push it right out through your mouth, making a really big 'Ha' sound from deep in your abdomen.

This releases tension in the face, jaw and upper body. It is also going to release a lot of negativity and anxiety in your body, because you're carrying that energy out of your body in a really big way with the out breath.

Note: Energising breathing exercises can cause you to become dizzy. Never carry out energising breathing exercises when driving or operating heavy machinery, sitting in traffic, or when you are in water. If you become dizzy, stop the exercise immediately and, if possible, lie down until the dizziness has completely passed.

Although it is an invigorating form of breathing, energising breathing is not the right technique to use after a long business lunch. A heavy meal, alcohol, and rapid breathing do not go well together. If you are feeling sleepy after lunch and want to clear your head before your next meeting, balancing breathing is a far more appropriate technique to use.

Balancing Breathing

Balancing breathing levels you out and brings you back into a state of equilibrium. Balancing breathing brings your breathing rate to around four to six breaths per minute.

With balancing breathing you really want to be breathing from your diaphragm, deep into your abdomen. In your mind's eye, try to focus on a point below your navel. This action massages the vagus nerve, which controls the nervous system. By using a restricted balancing breathing technique, you can really tone your nervous system down.

As the name suggests, balancing breathing techniques can be used at any time of the day or night without having any negative effects.

Exercise – Balancing Breathing

Four By Four Breathing

This is the simplest and easiest exercise you will learn. What amazes me is that so few people incorporate this into their lives. If you take nothing else from this book, this exercise – consistently practised three times a day – will have an incredibly beneficial effect on your life. It's hard for many people to fathom that something so simple can have such a big outcome. So many of my clients laugh when we practice this, but those same clients are the ones that consistently tell me how much this exercise has improved their wellbeing.

Method:

Sit still, with your back erect and your feet flat on the floor. Do not rest against the back of your chair. Have your hips level to the floor, and your knees at a ninety-degree angle. Rest your hands in your lap or on your thighs. You can have your eyes open or closed, but you will probably notice that your eyes will want to gently close after a period of time.

With your mind's eye focused on a point just below your navel, and imagining that your diaphragm is a jellyfish, breathe low and deeply into that point, at the same time imagining that your diaphragm jellyfish is gently moving down.

Breathe low and slow for a count of four. End with a very brief pause as your jellyfish diaphragm floats back up for an even count of four. Repeat this for at least four rounds. You can go for as long as you want, just keep your mind focusing on the gentle, slow, up and down motion of that jellyfish diaphragm, as it effortlessly floats through water.

This exercise works by imagining that your jellyfish diaphragm is 360 degrees round, and floating fully around your torso. Try to keep your upper chest and shoulders completely still. Most of the action is happening in your diaphragm.

If you've ever wanted to meditate and can't still the mind, or you've wanted a simple mindfulness practice, this is it. Use as required.

Calming Breathing

Calming breathing works in the same way as having a warm drink or a nightcap before bed. It knocks you out, or slows you down. For this reason, the technique used is quite different from energising and balancing breathing.

With calming breathing, you want to bring your breathing rate down to three breaths per minute or fewer, with a one-to-two ratio of breathing in and breathing out. If you find that you lose count, a good tip is to touch the pad of each fingertip against the pad of your thumb to count up to four on the in-breath, and then to cycle through this twice for a count of eight on the out-breath.

Be careful with calming breathing, as you really can slow yourself right down. It's not the right technique to use before going into a big meeting. Even if you're feeling a bit nervous, balancing breathing would be more appropriate before any kind of interaction with other people, as calming breathing can really put you to sleep and zone you out. NEVER practice this whilst driving, in water or during/before operating heavy machinery.

Calming breathing is the perfect technique to use when agitated. It helps you to calm down, switch off at the end of a busy day, or if the pressures of work are keeping you from getting a good night's rest. As such, this is ideally used prior to going to bed.

If possible, lie on your back to carry out calming breathing exercises. It's preferable to use nasal breathing on both the in-breath and the out-breath, but you may find it easier to control the out-breath if you exhale through your mouth, and this is fine if it works better for you.

Exercise – Calming Breathing

Four By Eight Ocean Sound Breathing

Method:

Lie comfortably flat and close your eyes. You may want to put a bolster, cushions or pillows under your knees. This takes the pressure off your kneecaps.

Now inhale slowly for a count of four. Briefly pause, then slowly exhale for a count of eight, emptying the air from the top of your chest all the way to the bottom of your abdomen. Repeat at least six times, slowly and consciously focusing internally on the breath.

These three exercises are the tip of the iceberg, and there are many variations on them. Don't confuse 'simple' with 'ineffective'. With these three simple exercises, you will be equipped to regulate your energy on demand when your body does not align to what your brain wants.

Key Takeaways

- The three main types of breathing are **energising breathing** (enlivening), **balancing breathing** (levelling), and **calming breathing** (relaxing).
- All three types of breathing are equally important, and support the different levels of awareness and alertness you need at different points throughout your working day.
- Through conscious breathing you are able to adjust the levels of CO_2 and oxygen in your body, and alter your ability to focus and relax.
- Simple is effective.

Chapter Five

Conscious Breathing Techniques For Your Business

It's hard to imagine that something as simple as breathing can help you in your business. However, it's often the really simple things in life that have the biggest impact. Being in control of your breath is a way that you can consciously take charge of the way you operate throughout your workday.

In the workplace there are a lot of energy vampires, whether it be people, situations that arise, meetings that you need to attend, there can be multiple things in the environment that drain your energy. Additionally, technology has made us dependent and lazy, which is unhealthy and unhelpful to your wellbeing.

The goal in this chapter is to learn some simple and effective techniques that can help you take control of your life in the workplace, freeing you from the energy vampires and releasing you from a dependence on technology.

Concentration

There is an expectation that we all have a linear level of concentration throughout the working day. However, human beings are simply not designed that way. We constantly shift between the sympathetic and parasympathetic nervous system taking a dominant role, with these shifts occurring every ninety minutes to three hours.

This means that there will be times during the working day when you really need to focus, and you're just not present and you can't get into it. As a result, you may either take far longer than necessary to complete a task, or procrastinate and take on other tasks that have less urgency and importance.

In both these instances, it can be easy to develop feelings of stress and anxiety about your inability to focus on the important task. This can quickly spiral into a cycle of disengagement.

The most important point to remember about concentration is that it's absolutely fine not to be able to stay fully focused for an eight-hour day. Some people can do it, but it's very rare, particularly if you're sitting all day. Sitting in one place for an extended period of time is very unnatural.

When you are seated behind a desk for hours on end it is very difficult to maintain core control and good posture. This, in turn, affects your ability to breathe efficiently. For this reason, a standing desk can be beneficial. However, it's not always possible to have a standing desk in your workplace.

This means that concentration, which will naturally ebb and flow due to shifts in the cycle of the sympathetic and parasympathetic nervous systems, can be even more greatly impacted, and may derail some of your success in business.

This is most often the case at those times when you just need to knuckle down and focus on the task at hand. You may be up against a tight deadline or working as part of a team, and so you need your concentration levels to be at their peak. If you are struggling to focus, this can be a big problem.

When this is the case, there are some really simple breathing techniques that you can do that will bring you into your body.

In The Workplace - Exercise
Take A Breather

The simplest strategy of all is to get up and move away from your computer. The act of moving away from your desk can be really impactful.

Take a deep breath in through your nose, and sigh out (you can exhale through your mouth). This is a conscious cue, telling your nervous system that everything is okay. It's a quick and simple 'reset and recalibrate' technique. Follow this with a few rounds of balancing breathing – in for four and out for four – through your nose. You can do this standing or seated somewhere other than your desk. If this is not practical, then doing this at your desk is fine.

When you return to your desk or the task at hand, place both feet flat on the floor, and sit upright with your butt pushed into the back of your chair. Your spine naturally curves into a slight 'S' shape, so you do not want to have the length of your spine pressed against the back of the chair, just your butt and your shoulders, if your chair back is high enough for this, and if it does not require you to push your shoulders back into an unnatural position.

The body responds really well to being in this position. When you are sitting upright, with your abdominal muscles relaxed and your chest open, so that you can breathe properly, you send a message to your nervous system that signals you are safe in your environment. Continue to breathe consciously, in and out, low and slow. Don't worry about counting, just breathe naturally.

When your body knows that you are safe and calm, it enables you to focus much more clearly. Practice this as often as needed during the day. Ideally, you want to schedule this at least every forty to sixty minutes.

Modern wearable technology has inbuilt reminders to help us consciously breathe. For example, my Apple watch has a 'breathe' app that reminds me to breathe throughout the day. You can set this for frequency and length of breath. I invite you to set up whatever cues you need to help you breathe consciously throughout the day. You don't need wearable technology to do this. Some simple cues include:

- On the half hour or the hour
- Five minutes before a meeting
- Immediately after a meeting
- Prior to (or after) a bathroom break
- Prior to (or after) a coffee or meal break
- Prior to opening your emails
- After a phone call
- As your computer or software is loading

Any other event or habit that happens during your day can act as a cue. By habit-stacking on regular cues, you will quickly and easily form this beneficial new habit.

What Goes Up Must Come Down

When concentration dips, it can be easy to go and grab a cup of tea or coffee, either with a couple of sugars in your drink or a couple of biscuits on the side. Or both. Although it may seem that this is an effective strategy to help you power through the next meeting or hit the next deadline, it actually really detracts from your ability to concentrate. This is because after the rush of the sugar and the caffeine there is an inevitable crash. What goes up must always come down, and this crash landing can be quite painful.

Conscious breathing, on the other hand, increases your energy and improves your levels of concentration without any detrimental effects. Unlike sugar or caffeine, where it is possible to have far too much, there are conscious breathing techniques - particularly those in the balancing breathing category - which can be used time and time again, whenever you need them.

In the workplace, there is often a lot of stuff going on around you which can be very distracting. Interruptions from phone calls, emails, and colleagues can make it very difficult to focus clearly, and really set you up for failure. It can be easy to blame yourself when you are unable to concentrate, but often the external stimuli of the workplace play a huge role. The same is true when you are working from home. In some ways, working from home can be more distracting.

Alongside sporadic interruptions, there can be workplace environmental problems that you need to contend with. These may include:

- poor lighting, which may be excessively bright or dim
- temperature, which may be excessively warm or cold
- air conditioning, which can be extremely dehydrating and noisy
- office conversations that you are not part of
- ringing phones
- technology, such as printers, scanners, and other devices that beep and bing throughout the day

No wonder it's difficult to concentrate! The good news is that by simply taking three or four minutes to carry out a balancing breathing exercise, at a measured pace, can bring yourself back into your body, and give yourself some control over your environment.

As we can be dependent on technology, think about ways you can control technology. Consider having scheduled times when you turn your emails and calendar off, have your phone on 'do not disturb', and log out of your social media accounts in order to minimise the interruptions to your work flow. These may be specific, set times during the day, or you may choose to do this at points where you have tight deadlines to meet or important proposals or presentations to write. Take it under your control, and breathe through the need to be constantly at the behest of technology.

Setting Small, Achievable Goals

Set yourself the goal of being completely focused for twenty minutes. After the twenty minutes is up, take a break and carry out a balancing breathing exercise, such as Box Breathing, for three to four minutes.

Once you have completed your balancing breathing exercise, fully focus on your work for another twenty minutes. By setting small, achievable goals you are likely to reach the larger milestones in a much shorter time frame.

In The Workplace - Exercise - Box Breathing

Sit calmly, with your feet flat on the floor and your hands resting in your lap. Inhale through the nose, low and deep, for four counts. Gently hold your breath at the top for four counts. Exhale gently for four counts. Hold your breath at the bottom for four counts. Visualise the jellyfish action of your diaphragm, as previously discussed – this helps you to picture the gentle flow of your breath as you practise this simple balancing exercise. Repeat this for at least four cycles.

Box breathing is one of the most common breathing techniques available. It is used by coaches, counsellors, yoga instructors, and

> breathwork practitioners, as a fast and effective way to help balance individuals. It is simple and effective. Of course, it only works if you practise it.

Later in the book, I will talk about how you can use box breathing as part of your workday.

Energy

As we have seen, energy is the new commodity, and breath is the engine that drives it. With this in mind, studies are showing that conscious breathing is a way to reenergise yourself, without the need to resort to stimulants such as drugs, caffeine, and sugar.

Energising breathing techniques are ideal when you need a 'pick-me-up' in the workplace. I do not recommend that you carry out these techniques for more than five rounds. Three rounds is sufficient for most people. You may come across other teachers who advocate long periods of an energising type of breath, and you may wish to explore that with those teachers. This may work for you. I believe that breathing techniques that are simple and easy to implement are the most effective.

First thing in the morning is the prime time for energising breathing. It may also be beneficial when you hit the mid-afternoon slump in the office.

There is evidence to show that food cravings only last for three to five minutes. Spending this amount of time following a balancing or energising breathing exercise (depending on how you are feeling), rather than reaching into the biscuit barrel or lolly jar, will give you a far more sustained release of energy than a sugary high provides.

If you still find that you are lacking in energy, three rounds of an energising breathing exercise will elevate your energy levels. Energising breathing always needs to be used with care. Overdoing it can induce anxiety, and may leave you feeling wired, rather than invigorated. For this reason, keep your energising breathing to a minimum, and don't use the technique beyond mid-afternoon, as it may be difficult to unwind at the end of the working day.

In The Workplace – Energising Exercise - Breath Of Fire

If you've ever done a yoga class, you may well know how to do Breath of Fire.

This is a really interesting breathing exercise, and although it can feel a little tricky if you've never done it before, it's well worth practicing. Holding your diaphragm in is not something that I often recommend, but in this instance, you're holding your stomach muscles, and exhaling from your belly.

Take three breaths in and out for a count of four on each inhale and exhale, then breathe in through your nose, pulling your abdomen in as you inhale. As you exhale, release the air in twenty short, sharp breaths, out through your nose, almost as though somebody's gently hitting you in the stomach.

Repeat for three rounds.

You don't have to worry about breathing in at all as your lungs will expand automatically as soon as you release that tension, and the air will automatically flow in, so you don't need to suck the air in. The focus of this exercise is on expelling the air in short, sharp, controlled breaths.

If you want to take this exercise up a notch - and this is often really good in the morning - you can do the same exercise, but on the second round of exhales, put your arms up in the air, either side of your head, as though you were about to do a pull-up, then, making fists with your hands, pull down repeatedly with each exhalation.

This will bring you into the present moment really quickly. So you do one round without the hands and then two rounds with the hands, then just let your breathing return to normal, and then you'll be incredibly energised.

Be warned, if you're wearing a lot of warm clothes, you'll get hot doing this exercise!

Note: Energising exercises can cause you to become dizzy. Never carry out energising breathing when driving or operating heavy machinery, sitting in traffic, or when you are in water. If you become dizzy, stop the exercise immediately and, if possible, lie down until the dizziness has completely passed.

Building Rapport

Have you ever been in a situation where you're talking to somebody, and you know that person is not present to you? How does that make you feel? How do you relate to that person? And what is the likelihood that the outcome of your interaction is going to be the best possible?

Think about the people you meet. The ones who are fully present with you are the ones you are more attracted to, and that you are more likely to interact with.

One of the techniques that you can use to really help build rapport, either with people you are meeting for the first time or those in the workplace, is to focus on looking them straight in the eye while breathing at a calm, measured pace, and adopting a relaxed, open posture that incorporates non-verbal cues such as nodding and smiling. Achieve this by using a balancing breathing technique - in and out through your nose for a count of four, low and slow. This calmness and presence is infectious, enabling you to take control and drive the conversation towards the outcome you are looking for.

If you find it confrontational to look people directly in the eye, as many people do, there is a really easy technique that you can use. Looking at the bridge of someone's nose, rather than looking straight into their eyes, is just as effective, and the other person will be unable to tell the difference.

In some cultures it is considered impolite to look people directly in the eye. If this is the case in your culture, or the culture of the person that you are speaking to, an alternative is to look at their mouth, so that you are still focusing your attention on what they are saying.

Breathing calmly while looking directly at someone, whether you are focusing on their eyes, the bridge of their nose, or their mouth, and nodding in response to what they are saying, means you can quickly build rapport with them.

Mirroring

There are lots of techniques for mirroring people's behaviour in order to put them at ease. However, this technique for building rapport focuses on displaying calm, confident behaviour that the other person can mirror. By being open and interested in the other person, they will tend to respond by mirroring your behaviour.

If the person that you are engaging with is finding it very difficult to be calm and measured, then focusing on your breathing for a simple count of four on the 'in' breath, and a count of four on the 'out' breath can be a very effective way of remaining calm. This applies in both face-to-face situations and on internet video call platforms.

When you are on a video call, rather than looking into the person's eyes, if you look into the camera it will appear to them as though you are looking directly at them. Apply the same techniques of breathing slowly and listening to them. Even through a screen people will pick up on a number of non-verbal cues. Be mindful of how you sit, and the use of your body language. Humans make constant judgements about another person's engagement through observing non-verbal cues.

A well-known and commonly used model for communication is known as the '7-38-55 rule'. These numbers represent percentages, which are allocated as follows: 7% is the spoken word, 38% is your tone of voice, and 55% is your body language. With this in mind, think of how much you are communicating through your body language, even on video conferencing.

As much of the communication that we have comes from non-verbal clues, breathing in a calm, measured way gives a really clear non-verbal signal that you are listening and attentive. It also shows your body to be calm and receptive. Intuitively, we can pick up on people who are not relaxed, calm, and open – try it for yourself next time you sense somebody is disengaged by focusing on which non-verbal cues you are picking up on.

Conscious breathing is also a great way to ensure you don't interrupt people. It is very easy to find yourself wanting to interrupt because you have something to say, or you want to respond to what they are saying. Building rapport means holding onto the understanding that most people's favourite topic of conversation is themselves. By listening to them and applying the 80/20 rule, so that they speak for eighty per cent of the time and you speak for twenty per cent of the time, you will quickly make a connection.

It can sometimes be quite difficult to do this, and so using a calm, measured balancing breathing technique when the other person is talking helps you to concentrate and listen to what they are saying, rather than wanting to respond in a reactive way. Being proactive in the way you engage allows your reactivity to calm down.

It can sometimes feel as though you need to respond immediately to each and every point that someone raises. In reality, you won't forget the things that are really important. And even if you do, they will almost certainly come up again at a later point in time.

This means that you can focus on your breathing and your non-verbal cues to acknowledge the other person. This helps you to build a high level of engagement with people. Many people in the workplace don't do this, because they are already focused on the next thing they need to do. No matter how busy you are, though, when you are speaking with someone, you need to be fully present with that person. Conscious breathing helps you to be fully present to the situation you are in.

If you truly don't have time to speak to that person at that moment, this is fine. It is important to meet your own needs. You can do this by quietly and clearly explaining why you are not able to talk at that time, and acknowledging that you do want to talk to them at a time when you can give them your full attention. Being realistic about what you can provide to people is much more helpful to you and to them.

Conflict Resolution

As human beings, no matter where we are, we bring our full suite of emotions to every situation. Obviously this will include the workplace, and it stands to reason that, as humans, those around you may get angry from time to time.

We've all seen it, when people want to get others to see things their way, so that they can get what they want., Tthis is not always done in a resourceful manner. Ultimately, we are all human, and no one is perfect. This means that some people can push back hard, in a way that is often harsh. The desire to be right all the time and to be 'the winner' can be strong for many people. It's the whole Western 'might is right' approach to life.

When you are in conflict with colleagues, listening is the most powerful way to resolve the situation. You don't need to like what they are saying. You don't need to like their tone of voice or the dictatorial and blaming language they are using. That's all fine. What you do need to do is protect your space. You can do this by being in your body and being fully present. In this way, you can let the other person get all of their anger out.

By breathing in a measured way, being respectful, nodding, asking questions when appropriate, and acknowledging what the person is saying, you can greatly reduce your reactions. You can't always change the way other people think and behave, but your state of being is something you can control. Over time, and with practice, by using balancing breathing techniques in conflict situations, you can change the course of the conversation. You also reduce your reactions to others' behaviour, thereby reducing your own stress levels.

By calmly breathing, being fully present with the other person, and listening to what they have to say, it is far easier to resolve conflict. Whether or not you agree with what they have to say, that's their reality. It's their story. Being respectful to them and allowing them to tell you their story without being attached to an outcome can be really empowering for you. When you don't go down into the rabbit hole with them and react to everything they are saying, you free yourself.

Sometimes, people just need to get things off their chest. You just happen to be the person they are directing it at. It is always good to consider the other person's intent. It might feel as though they are attacking you, but it is very hard to attack someone who is calm and present, and who is acknowledging you.

Being calm and present allows you to be more measured, thoughtful, and impactful. This is because, as you consciously breathe, you are giving yourself the space, in your body and in your mind, to respond in a more appropriate way. When you are really riled up, it is easy to say stupid things which you later regret.

When people come to you in a high-conflict situation, by breathing and listening until they have got absolutely everything out that they need to get out, you can change the entire narrative. It also enables you to feel better about the situation, because you're not agitated and reactive.

The more you practice this, the easier it becomes. Using breathing techniques enables you to create a break point between the time you would normally react and when you actually respond. This means it is likely you will be a little kinder and more thoughtful in your approach.

You don't have to win all the time. In fact, by engaging in conflict, you automatically lose. You can listen to other people's views and you can present your own views in a way that is calm and respectful. By being conscious and aware in your own body, you help yourself and those around you.

Many people who are aggressive and angry are coming from a place of fear, lack, or uncertainty. They are reacting because their worldview isn't being supported, and so they lash out at other people. Nothing is ever gained by being aggressive - particularly in the workplace.

Using your breath as a tool to be present enables you to make a mindset shift and look after your own state of being. This means that things are immediately better - for you and for others. Giving other people the opportunity to be truly heard means that you have the best chance of truly helping to solve their problems, in a way that is not detrimental to you.

Agreeing to disagree is fine. It is important to understand that when you, or someone else, begins to get hot and red in the face, this is a signal of a shift to the sympathetic nervous system. By ensuring that more blood reaches the muscles in order to provide them with oxygen, the body is preparing to take fight or flight action. As a result, the blood vessels in the face also expand, increasing blood flow.

When you are in a state of stress, you increase your risk of physical and mental health problems. When your sympathetic nervous system is in control, it is much more difficult to think rationally. By being in your body and protecting your state of wellbeing, you are able to ensure there are better outcomes to any conflict situations that arise in the workplace, to the benefit of everybody.

Changing The Course Of Conversations

Being calm and measured can change other people's state of being. When you look at the great leaders, such as the Dalai Llama and Nelson Mandela, people are drawn to them because they are very calm and fully present. Think about the people in your life who exude confidence, and I am sure you will see that they come from a place of calm and quiet strength.

Anybody can achieve this - being fully present in a conversation enables you to be in control of the environment around you. Ensuring other people feel heard and understood gives you the space to have them reflect on other points of view. By breathing in a measured fashion, you can do this in a way that is not aggressive, threatening, rigid, or challenging.

This takes practice. It doesn't happen overnight. Becoming aware of your own reactions and letting go of the need to be right is key. Using conscious breathing techniques to bring yourself into the present moment whenever you notice negative thoughts and feelings arising releases you from reacting to other people's views and opinions.

The reality is that the vast majority of people on the planet do not agree with everything you think. Everyone has their own individual point of view that has been formulated through all of their experiences.

More often than not, when people are very agitated it is because they have come to that conversation with a problem. Where possible, once you have heard and understood the problem, you can then offer solutions. People generally respond very well to solutions-based thinking. If you are not able to provide a solution, by being present and aware, you can ask really good questions. By being genuinely interested in their answers, you can then develop a greater understanding and may be able to find the solution together.

Key Takeaways

- When you are struggling to focus, by using simple breathing techniques to bring yourself back into your body you can improve your levels of concentration.
- Breathing in a calm, measured way gives a really clear non-verbal signal that you are listening to the other person, and that you are interested in what they have to say.
- Using your breath as a tool to be present enables you to make a mindset shift, look after your own state of being, and help solve other people's problems in a way that is not detrimental to you.

Braith runs an eight-week results programme for individuals looking to make significant change in their life.

Take the first step by getting in touch with Braith at: https://braithbamkin.com.au/

Chapter Six

Mindset

Mindset and mindfulness are buzzwords at the moment. All too often people tell you that you need to have a mindset of positivity, but they don't give you the tools that enable you to achieve this shift.

Conscious breathing can really help you to create this mindset of positivity, and the power to be fully present. The purpose of using conscious breathing for business is to achieve your **desired future state**. It is about creating a shift from where you are to where you want to be.

Your desired future state may be a short-term goal, such as becoming calm and focused within the next hour so that you can give a great presentation, or it may be a longer-term goal, such as changing the way you communicate with other people in the workplace.

Whatever the goal, the purpose of conscious breathing is to develop an understanding of your current state and an awareness of your desired future state, and to make the shift from one to the other.

It is possible to make these shifts because your personality isn't fixed. You change and adapt as you move through different stages of your life. The way you look at your life changes. This is because life is dynamic.

Mastering Your Reactions

Through my work as a BNI Executive Director, I have been able to closely observe what sets successful people apart from those who find things more of a struggle. Over the years, I have learned that people who have mastery over the way they react to external stimuli are more successful. Mastery over the way you react comes through being connected to yourself.

Being aware of your breath is the gateway to being conscious in your behaviour. It is, to a great extent, a process of unlearning much of what was absorbed during childhood, when the adult world imposed an unnatural framework over healthy, natural behaviours and modes of being.

For instance, babies naturally breathe from their diaphragms and have an innate understanding of how to self-soothe. All of this changes around the time we start school, at which point children begin to move into learned behaviours which affect us unconsciously.

We have layers and layers of these unconscious behaviours that prevent us from breathing in the way we were designed to breathe. When you unlearn these behaviours, and relearn how to breathe in the way your body intuitively wants to breathe, it becomes easy. You achieve this through developing a greater awareness of yourself.

It's very easy to act unconsciously. In the workplace or in your day-to-day life, if you are looking for a desired future state that is different from your current state, you are going to have to consciously change how you react to things that are going on around you.

The only person who can make that change is you. We all have to take responsibility for ourselves.

When you make the decision to take responsibility, you create the possibility of change. Conscious breathing brings you into your body, connects you to yourself, and creates a circuit breaker so that you can consciously change your behaviour.

Creating A Circuit Breaker

It is very easy to drive on autopilot - particularly on familiar routes. We know that we need to pay attention and have a high level of awareness of our surroundings, but many people switch to automatic. It's the same in the workplace. We can find ourselves going through the motions, distracting ourselves by checking emails and looking at social media, until before you know it, it's time for your coffee break. You wander down to the break room, have a coffee with your colleagues, and stroll back to your desk at eleven o' clock. Only to find that you've done nothing. The same can be true when working from home. In many cases we have even more distractions at home.

Energising Exercise - Bellows Breathing

Start your day with three rounds of this energising breath. An energising breath consists of any practise with thirty-plus breaths per minute. This slightly reduces the CO_2 in your system, and very slightly increases your blood O_2 levels.

Bellows Breathing gets its name from the action of the rapid in and out movement of your diaphragm - like a pair of bellows stoking a fire. You need to be sitting in a comfortable position. You can stand, if you want, but do not lie down for this practise. Just be mindful that bellows breathing may sometimes leave you lightheaded, so if you are standing, be aware of this possibility. Hence my view that a seated position is best.

Have your spine upright, and imagine the bellows in your diaphragm – almost as though someone was punching you in the stomach, and you contract in reaction, in a short, sharp manner, and breathing out in an equal forced manner. Your diaphragm is going in and out like a pair of bellows, with one 'in and out' per second. This is quite rapid.

Do this for a count of thirty cycles, rest for three to five normal inhalations, then repeat a further two times, or up to a maximum of five in total.

After you have completed your bellows breathing, you will feel energised and alive. This is why I recommend this exercise as your first morning ritual.

Note: Energising exercises can cause you to become dizzy. Never carry out energising breathing when driving or operating heavy machinery, sitting in traffic, or when you are in water. If you become dizzy, stop the exercise immediately and, if possible, lie down until the dizziness has completely passed.

The above exercise is a healthy alternative to reaching for your phone the moment you wake up, checking your emails and messages from clients, and responding immediately.

Whether you are distracting yourself throughout the day, or diving straight into work the moment you wake up, you're in an unconscious pattern of behaviour. Conscious breathing can give you the break you need to take control of the way in which you react to your work environment. You can turn notifications off to avoid distractions, and you can ensure that when people are asking you for things in their timeframe that you take a breath and then respond in a way that is appropriate to your needs. Is it appropriate to meet their requirements in their time frame? What is your timeframe? What is appropriate for you?

All too often people overcommit and agree to do things that are going to put them under a great deal of pressure. The alternative reaction is to shoot off a plethora of reasons why they can't do the task they have been asked to carry out. Either way, the outcome is not positive, leading to feelings of resentment, stress, and being undervalued.

If you find yourself in a situation like this, step back and take a deep, slow breath into your belly, and a slow, gentle inaudible release through your nose. I refer to this as a 'circuit-breaker breath', as this simple act gives you a split second break to make a decision that is going to be much more appropriate and beneficial to everyone involved.

By acting consciously in the workplace you can develop immunity to the external pressures that people place on you. You can take control of your own life. This works equally well in your personal life, particularly with your life partner.

Other useful places to practice this breath are on phone calls dealing with frustrating people or on Zoom calls. In other words, this is a really simple circuit breaker, useful for many life situations.

NB: when taking this circuit breaker breath, it's very important not to accompany it with negative body language or an infantile 'huff'.

Recognising Choice

Life is a continuous act of making choices. Each choice has an outcome, and you are in control of the outcome.

It is easy to act on autopilot. We can go through

life letting it happen to us, or we can be the controller of our own world.

Think about a time when you have just been going through the motions of life. How did that feel for you? Did you find that you made the best life decisions? Humans are designed to have a negativity bias. We are primed to react to, and store, negative stimuli. In the workplace, this means people can be extremely aware of the negative things that are going on around them, and all too often the reaction is to personalise those things, even when it is not personal.

For instance, if you have twenty amazing things happen to you in the workplace over the course of a day, and in addition to those amazing things one really bad thing happens, what are you going to spend the evening thinking about? It's very likely to be the one bad thing. Because the negativity bias pushes you towards that outcome. You are programmed to hold onto problems.

However, there is a choice. You can take a negative scenario and reframe it. In any situation, each of the people involved will have their own story. You can choose to hold on to your story, you can take on other people's stories, or you can choose not to react at all.

The belief systems that we create, about ourselves and the people around us, can have a massive impact on the way we go about our work day. When you then layer this with the stress of poor postural habits, poor breathing habits, and negativity bias, you can find yourself in a situation where you have become your own worst enemy. It's very hard to then break out of that cycle.

Conscious breathing gives you a little bit of space in your everyday life to look at a situation for what it actually is. The story that you tell yourself about the person at work who is being demanding or aggressive is almost certainly not a reflection of what is actually going on in their life.

When we keep building these beliefs, it creates a foundation that can have a dramatic impact on our personality. If people at work are constantly giving you negative messages because they are so caught up in their own stress and anxiety, it can begin to generate an unrealistic, negative perception of who you are. At this point, it is easy to begin attracting more of the same.

Exercise – Highs and Lows

Think about your last week at work. What were the highs? What were the lows? Chances are, you could think about more low points than highlights. What was your contribution to those low points (be honest with yourself)? What could you have done differently that may have generated a different outcome? How could you have used a circuit-breaker breath or balanced breathing to contribute to that different outcome?

Now think about the highlights of the week. What was going on for you around those situations? How were you feeling? And more importantly, how were you being? By using some of the techniques in this book, I'd like to invite you to reframe and take control of what could be a negative situation, and turn it into a positive outcome. This takes practise. A consistent conscious breathing practise will help, but it needs to be regular and applied.

The Law Of Attraction

If you ever look at people around you in the workplace and wonder why the good stuff always happens to them, then you have an unrealistic and negative perception of yourself, which becomes a self-fulfilling prophecy. If other people always seem to be getting promotions, winning awards, receiving praise, and being chosen for exciting projects, while you're always stuck on the side lines, then you are almost certainly experiencing problems with the law of attraction.

When you give yourself positive messages you create a positive energy. Other people are naturally attracted to positivity. So when you are able to let go of your negative self-talk, and not absorb or personalise the stress and anxiety that people around you are generating, you develop a positive outlook which then attracts more positive experiences.

Your body is made up of energy. You produce an electromagnetic field, and people can feel this energy. When we talk about people having good vibes or feel that there's something we don't like about another person, we are picking up on their energy. We all put out an energy, and we all pick up on each other's energy.

If the energy that you put out is that you're ok, that you're confident, and that you're positive, then people will pick up on this. Conscious breathing puts you into a state where you are calm and confident, and people are highly attracted to this.

If you are in a situation in the workplace where you feel that you keep getting passed over and you react to this in a negative way, then you're going to keep getting passed over. Being positive doesn't mean being a doormat and saying yes to everything that people want you to do. Being assertive is part of being positive, and part of putting out a good energy.

If you are really clear about what is and isn't ok, then people will respond to that. Most people who are not able to achieve their desired future state are really unclear about what it is that they want. They know that they are not happy with how things are in the present, but they don't know what they want things to look like in the future.

When you're not connected to yourself and fully present, you become stressed, tense, judgemental, angry, or physically ill. None of these things is helpful when you want to build a successful career.

Everything becomes centred on problems rather than solutions. Think about times in your life when this has happened to you. Again, I'm sure it will correlate to when you have been living life on autopilot.

Downward Spirals or Outward Ripples?

Life is not always going to unfold the way you would like it to. It's our reactions to life that will determine how we are impacted.

Reacting in a negative way when someone drops their stuff on you is only going to affect you. Often people completely forget about what they've said or done a short time later (I'm certainly one of those people, as my partner reminds me). However, if you choose to carry that stuff with you for the rest of the day, then drag it home and carry it around some more, you will feel increasingly angry and resentful. This is going to affect your digestion and your breathing, which in turn will affect your sleep. So then you will wake up the following morning not feeling rested, you'll be tired at work, so you'll be more hunched over, which will affect your breathing and your energy levels, which then impacts your work, so another shit-bomb gets dropped on you, and the downward spiral continues.

On the other hand, when you are calm, joyful, and able to think clearly, you are able to see solutions. People respond to this, and it creates an outward ripple where the workplace becomes increasingly harmonious, productive, and solutions-driven.

Conscious breathing really gives you a roadmap to get out of this cycle. Taking responsibility for your own state of being means having awareness of what your desired future state of being is. If you can't visualise this clearly then how are you going to move towards it?

When you have a clear vision of where you want to go then you begin to see the things that will take you there. This is very different to having aspirations, where you simply desire a bigger house or a better job or a higher income. This kind of thinking puts you in a mindset of lack. Rather than thinking very specifically about how you want your life to be, so that you can then become aware of the steps that will take you there, if you focus on the things you don't have, how can you attract anything to yourself?

Consciously breathing for just five minutes a day can take you into a very similar space as meditation. It stops the negative feedback loop between the brain and the body. By using a couple of very simple breathing exercises you quickly see that things are not as you had perceived them when you were caught in a negative spiral.

If you believe that life is hard, and you keep giving yourself that feedback, then life is going to be hard. If you tell yourself that your job is unrewarding, that no one appreciates you, that the people around you are all incompetent, and that nothing gets done properly unless you do it yourself, you are feeding that negative brain/body feedback cycle over and over again with negative messages.

Developing a positive attitude is crucial to your success. Your mind is yours. Your thought process is the only thing you have genuine choice in. For this reason, your mindset is the most valuable thing that you have.

Mindset is the difference between moving through life with relative ease, and being in a place of constant struggle. You need to be conscious of the problems and challenges that exist, on a personal and a global level. It's also crucially important to be aware of the incredible, positive advances that are taking place, both personally and globally.

Exercise – Commitment To Practice

Earlier in the book, I taught you how to use box breathing. I now want you to commit to five minutes of box breathing every day. I suggest using this earlier in your day – put it in your diary and make it a non-negotiable part of your routine.

Some suggestions to make it easier to incorporate this into your life are to habit stack the exercise with something you do regularly, such as a coffee break or lunch, or around your bathroom breaks or hydration breaks. Other great places to do this is when you are waiting for a Zoom meeting to happen, waiting for meeting participants to arrive in a physical space, or if you are ever waiting outside someone's office for a meeting to start, including medical appointments.

If you catch public transport to work, this is also a great place to practise box breathing. Before you know it, you will be doing this several times every day, and you will notice a difference in your life. It usually takes a couple of weeks.

I like to have a coffee mid-morning. It usually takes three to five minutes to make, and I use box breathing during this time. I did teach you to do this exercise seated, but once you get the hang of it, you can do it standing in a comfortable posture, with your eyes open but not fixed on any particular object.

What I like most about this exercise is that I don't automatically reach for my phone and start mindlessly engaging with social media or emails. If I'm by myself, sitting in a café, I will try to box breathe for the duration of my coffee. It's quite a liberating feeling, not being tied to your phone. However, I am human, and don't always nail this!

A word of caution - do not practise this while you are driving.

Owning Your Mindset

Have you ever noticed that there seem to be two types of people? Those who feel that they cannot take action until... and they will fill in this blank with a million different things. Then there is the other type of people - those who take action, regardless of what is going on, so that they can take as much responsibility as possible for influencing the outcome.

Whether you are a business owner or an employee, taking control of your mindset and your circumstances is crucial. When you own your mindset, amazingly positive things can come out of extremely negative situations.

For instance, I bought my first house in the middle of a recession. Everyone said that I was crazy, but I could see the benefits of making that choice at that time. During times of adversity, people do amazing things to change and improve their circumstances. You make a choice as to whether the world is going to shape you, or you're going to shape your world.

On a broader scale, Nelson Mandela is a truly inspirational example of someone who owned their mindset. I visited Robben Island, where he was imprisoned for twenty-seven years, and it is extraordinary. Mandela lived in a tiny box, and when he wasn't locked up he was breaking rocks in the limestone quarry. When they drove us out to the quarry the white rocks were so blinding that I could hardly see. And even though it was a cold day, the sun reflecting off the rocks raised the temperature in the quarry until it was as hot as hell.

Yet here was a man who became the president of his country, and did it with love and compassion. He became one of the world's greatest leaders. Because he never let his mind get taken over by the people who wanted to oppress him. It's all about choice.

Shifting Your Focus

The key is to start connecting to yourself, and giving yourself space - space on the inside, to create better frameworks, to understand what you want, and to make better decisions. Space to become solutions-focused. Stop thinking about all the things you don't want and start getting clarity about what you do want. Everything you want is already there. The world is abundant. You can look at it for all the lack, or you can look at it for all the abundance.

Focus on the acts of random kindness, and become part of that network. At the moment the hot word is 'pivot'. If you're not in the right mindset, you can't pivot. This is because in order to pivot, you have to be open to change.

Ultimately, it's easier to be happy than it is to be miserable. It takes far less energy. Being unhappy is draining, and it makes life hard. The truth is that life doesn't need to be a struggle. This doesn't mean there won't be challenges, but the way you relate to those challenges really dictates how the world reacts to you.

Become conscious of the actions, the language, and the mindset that supports you. Don't look for faults, in yourself or others. Seek understanding. Once you have connected with yourself, you can begin to connect with other people in a much more meaningful, productive, and helpful way.

We are all looking for certainty, but it doesn't exist. By developing a mindset that accepts change as an intrinsic part of life, so that you can let go of trying to control everything, you free yourself from constantly battling against the world. You can't stop the changes that are going to come. But you can learn to take a deep breath and see the benefits that they bring.

In The Workplace – Case Study - Sarah - Anxiety And Fear

Sarah was a very anxious person. All through her life, people had told her that she had a lot of anxiety, and so she started to believe that this was true, and she began to display those behaviours.

She was quite timid, uptight, and afraid that people were going to judge her. When situations that she wasn't familiar with came up in her life, she felt very uncomfortable. As a result, she never volunteered to do anything over and above her role.

After many years working for the same company, she was asked to take on a more senior role. She decided that she really wanted to take the new role, but realised that if she was going to be successful, she would need to address her anxiety.

She realised that every time she was confronted with a new situation she would go into a very fast, shallow breathing pattern. She came to me and explained that she had anxiety.

As she was consistently breathing shallow and high in her chest she was triggering her sympathetic nervous system. This was continually putting her into a fight or flight scenario, signalling to her brain and body that she was stressed. Although she understood the problems, she just wasn't able to calm herself down.

One of the requirements of the new role was that she would need to run meetings with a small team. She knew that she was capable of doing this, but her physical fear and anxiety were holding her back.

As a result, she wanted to learn some techniques that would help her to regulate her breathing and reduce her anxiety. We started with some balancing breathing exercises that she could use before meetings.

We tried a simple technique, breathing in for a count of four, and out for a count of eight. At first, this was too much for Sarah, and so we reduced the count to breathing in for a count of three and out for a count of six. Provided you are doubling the length of time you exhale, compared to the amount of time you inhale, this technique will be very calming.

Sarah quickly found that by calming herself down before meetings, she was able to step into these situations with a clarity that she hadn't previously had. She began using this breathing technique in all sorts of situations that she found confronting.

We started adding more calming breath exercises. In particular, she found the humming breath to be very useful, as it seemed to calm her quickly. We also started adding balancing breathing (box breathing and alternate nostril breathing) as part of her daily routine.

Through incorporating balancing breathing into her daily life, she found a presence of mind that she hadn't had before. She started to notice that she was able to listen to people better, and that she could engage more effectively with people in her workplace.

Before long, she began to be viewed as being extremely competent in her new role. She realised that she was enjoying the meetings, and that she was achieving a lot.

She was doing so well that she got asked to deliver a presentation. Once again, her anxiety came to the fore, and she became very nervous about getting up on stage.

She knew that she would need a lot of energy in order to get through the speech, and so she came back to me and we added in an energising breathing technique, called Breath of Fire (see page 115), in order to get her into the right frame of mind, and then went over the balancing breathing techniques, so that when she stepped out on stage she was able to use her breathing to regulate the pattern of her speech, and sustain her energy for the entire presentation.

Many people speak very fast when they're on stage, but by practicing how to use the in breath and out breath, and how to take pauses, Sarah found that as she moved through her speech, there were points in the presentation where she could naturally stop and take a slow, gentle breath in and a slow, gentle breath out.

Using this technique, she felt she was in control of the room. She made a few mistakes and fumbled a few words, but after she got off stage she was delighted that she had been speaking competently and confidently for forty minutes, even though she'd never spoken on stage before.

People were amazed and impressed, telling her that they had always thought of her as being the nervy one, but that they really loved her talk. Her success with this presentation gave her the confidence to start volunteering to give more presentations, take on more project work, and to sit on committees.

She still got anxious and nervous sometimes, but because she had the tools to bring herself back into her body, she was able to manage her anxiety and let her confidence shine through.

A lot of people who are anxious and nervous aren't fully present. Sarah learned that by breathing slowly through the nose and focusing on the other person, she was able to have really honest and connected conversations.

At first she felt that she couldn't look people in the eyes, so I taught her the technique of looking at people between the eyebrows, just above the bridge of the nose. I explained that when you use this technique, it's important that you don't stare at this point in a completely fixed and unmoving way. You need to nod, and use gestures and feedback that acknowledges the person you are talking to.

Sarah had previously avoided a lot of one-to-one conversations. But she now blossomed, and built her team into the highest performing team in the business.

Behavioural Activation Theory

Although it may feel as though you cannot change your thoughts and feelings, you can have a big effect on your emotions and outlook. One of the ways in which this can take place is through Behavioural Activation Theory, which I first studied as part of my undergraduate psychology degree, and have used to great effect in my life ever since.

Behavioural Activation Theory is perhaps most easily understood as 'fake it till you make it'. Essentially, if you believe that you are happy, you will be happy. A good example of how Behavioural Activation Theory works can be seen in facial-feedback hypothesis, which is founded on the idea that your facial expressions signal emotions to your brain, through the contraction of particular muscles, as well as to other people, through visual cues. So if you are frowning you will feel emotions such as sadness, and if you are smiling, you will feel emotions such as happiness. When the particular muscles that create certain expressions are in use, your mind is unable to separate the use of those muscles from the associated emotion.

If you adopt a happy expression then your brain, and the people around you, will perceive you as being happy. This perception will result in more favourable responses from people around you, which in turn will help to ensure you attract more happiness into your life.

We've talked about how your energy can affect the world around you. This is another illustration of how people respond to your state of being. Science has shown that being in a state of gratitude, which is often characterised in popular culture as having an open and loving heart, means that you cannot be concurrently sad.

The fastest way to get into this state of gratitude, which in turn will trigger your behavioural state (ie: gratitude manifests as a smiling, open face) – this activates a feedback loop, and can very quickly change your state, and the way people relate to you - is to pause and inhale low and slow into your abdomen. Use either a balancing breath technique or, if you are particularly agitated, start with a calming breath technique, as outlined earlier in the book.

Behaviour Activation Theory

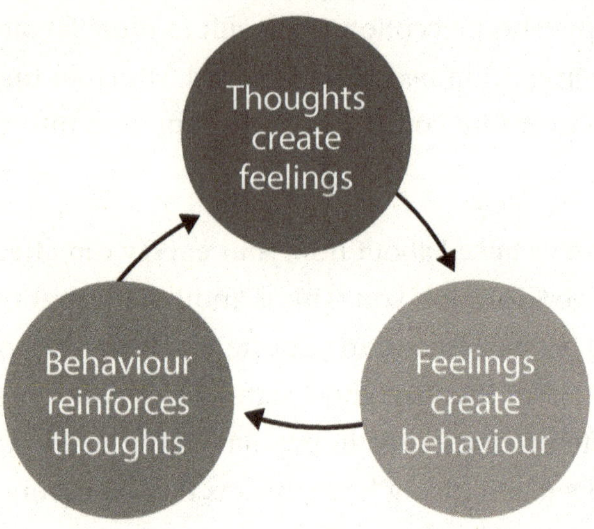

In life, and particularly in your working environment, (including online meetings) remember one of the main ways others read your mood is through your facial expressions. If you look grumpy, stressed, and tired, and this is what the people around you see, then they will treat you accordingly. If you look happy and calm then people will react to you based on the perception that this is how you feel, creating a positivity loop.

Through conscious breathing you can become very centred and focused, and those around you will respond to this. If you want to change your external environment then you need to start by changing your internal environment.

Key Takeaways

- Conscious breathing helps you to develop an understanding of your current state and an awareness of your desired future state, so that you can make the shift from one to the other.
- Your thought process is the only thing you have genuine choice in. For this reason, your mindset is paramount.
- Connecting to yourself, and giving yourself space to create better frameworks, helps you to understand what you want and enables you to make better decisions.

Chapter Seven

Less is More

When I was first in the workplace in the eighties, I remember when our office got its first fax machine. As the first test fax came into the office that day, twenty of us stood around the clunky 'state of the art' machine watching it slowly (and it was very slow) deliver a piece of thermo-printed paper. We were all in awe of this amazing technology, and I remember us talking about how the workplace was going to change forever, and that humans would get to spend so much more time in leisure, and these machines would do our work for us.

Fast-forward to the twenty-first century, and nothing could be further from the truth. In contemporary Western culture, there seems to be a belief that being really busy is a marker of success. Getting into work early, staying late, working through lunch, working weekends, taking calls and doing work on holidays, are all culturally acceptable, and in many cases expected work habits.

The lack of delineation between work and leisure that has been brought about by rapid advances in technology, and the need for immediacy that is an expectation of the modern workplace, makes it very difficult for many of us to say no, and to stop work. Workers and business owners alike wear their multi-tasking and long work hours like a badge of honour, and yet it is slowly creating many stressed and sick individuals.

I would like to invite you to think about creating a healthy relationship with work. It is good to do less, and to take time out for yourself. This does not make you a failure. Conscious breathing during your day is a tool that can give you the space you need.

Adding one energising breathing session into your morning routine, then taking the time to carry out one balancing breathing session during the working day, and winding down with a calming breathing session before bed is all you need. Practice this consistently for a few weeks, and you will definitely feel a shift.

Do You Own A Business Or Do You Own A Job?

The idea of the four-hour work week was the big thing a few years ago, and if this is an option for you then that's great. However, working just four hours a week is not something that it possible for everyone. Many business owners get caught in a trap, where, rather than owning a business, they own a job.

If you are working in and on your business all the time, there will always be things that need to be managed. It takes a big shift in mindset to own your business, rather than your business owning you.

Successful business ownership means that it is possible to leave your business for a month or two while you go off and do something else. If it is not possible for you to do this, and instead you are inundated with demands every time you turn your back, then the reality is that you are selling time for money.

All too often, the business owners who are really stressed and who find their businesses really challenging are those people who have the 'employee of their own business' mindset.

The same is true for employees, in a slightly different way. If you are constantly chasing promotions, bonuses, raises, and accolades, then you can easily find yourself taking on far more than is reasonable or practical in order to achieve your goals. In this instance, it is really important to have a beginning, a middle, and an end to your working day, with strict boundaries about what you take on.

Creating Healthy Boundaries

Whether you are a business owner or an employee, setting boundaries is crucial. So many people are not clear about what they want, and as a result they attempt to be good at everything, which is not possible.

For this reason, having a 'less is more' mentality can help you to be really successful, as it enables you to gain clarity and focus, so that you can put your energy into the things that are going to move you forward, rather than simply running in circles.

The feeling of being in overwhelm, and of being in a state of perpetual motion, sets you up for more of the same. When you think about how you want your future to be, it probably doesn't involve being in overwhelm.

I am a big advocate of having a daily meditation practice, but I know that many people find sitting in meditation difficult. One of the great things about conscious breathing is that it is a shortcut to being present, and if you're somebody who can't meditate, this is a great alternative. You don't need to learn how to meditate for hours at a time, you can simply consciously breathe for a few minutes a day and create an amazingly strong connection with yourself.

Being calm, in control, and not overworked, is an environment you can create for yourself. Being scared that you are going to lose your business or your job if you say 'no' to anything is ultimately self-defeating. If you take on so much that you cannot give the appropriate level of time, energy, and attention to your tasks, you often end up creating more problems than you solve.

Learning how to put boundaries around your time is crucial. With the shift to so many people working from home, the divisions between personal time and work have become even fuzzier. The daily commute has been replaced by a minute's walk to the study, and that extra time at the desk is often now filled with more work.

With the shift from the workplace to our homes, the belief that people would be less productive has proved to be unfounded. Instead, there is a recognition that we don't need to create a reality where we are permanently stressed and tired.

Achieving Optimum Performance

Finding the balance, and connecting to yourself through your breathing, is a little like driving a manual car. Instead of driving down the freeway at 100 kilometres an hour in first gear with the engine screaming, you can cruise down the freeway in fifth gear, doing far less damage and with much less effort. You can still get there in first gear, but it puts a lot more stress on the engine.

Performing in an optimum way allows you to achieve a great deal without it feeling stressful and overwhelming, because you are focused. It's like in a superhero film, when you see through the superhero's eyes. Even though in reality everything is moving fast, to the superhero it is as though time has slowed right down. They can see exactly what's coming and what they need to do in order to solve the problems they are facing.

Being connected to yourself enables you to see things for what they really are and to control the environment around you much more effectively. Conversely, when your sympathetic nervous system is continually getting signals that you're stressed, you lose sight of the world around you, and it looks as though everything is hurtling towards you in the most out of control way.

Thinking Small

There are always going to be stressful situations that need dealing with. That's just part of life. Sometimes you will not be able to avoid late nights and early mornings in order to get things done. However, being centred, so that you are fully present, means you will be able to manage those stressful times far better, and to see that they have a beginning, a middle, and an end. This means that you know you can deal with it.

When you have a beginning, a middle, and an end, you can break things down into smaller pieces. Take the example of working out at the gym. If you have to do three sets of twelve reps each, rather than simply counting from one to twelve through each set, you can break those reps down, into six, then three, then two, then one, until before you realise it, you're done. And the process is made so much easier by breathing into it.

Key Takeaways

- Taking on too many responsibilities can weigh you down and hold you back, rather than helping you to move forward.
- When you are calm and connected to yourself, you create an environment that you can control.
- Breaking things down into smaller pieces, with a beginning, a middle, and an end to every goal, ensures you can achieve your desired future state with far less effort.

Chapter Eight

Posture

Dr Belisa Vranich, author of Breathe: Fourteen Days To Oxygenating, Recharging, And Refuelling Your Body And Brain, and one of my go-to experts and mentors in the world of awakened breathing, once told me that she believes the three things that prevent us from premature aging are being able to squat with ease, twist with comfort, and breathe naturally.

All too often, our diaphragm does not move easily and naturally. Years of bad habits and poor breathing technique can mean that when you are in this disconnected state, your thoracic cavity may feel seized up, and preclude you from being able to twist and breathe naturally (your body wants to breathe the way it was designed to, we just get in its way sometimes). Not using your muscles correctly can cause your thoracic cavity to lock into position. If you think of your thoracic cavity as being like a cage, and your lungs as being like balloons, then when the balloons are inflating and deflating, if the cage around them isn't flexible, so that you haven't got the room to inflate the balloons, it's going to cause you problems.

Your posture has a massive impact on the way you breathe. In the workplace, you may be using furniture that is not ergonomically designed and hunching over your computer in a way that pushes your head forward. Working from home can exacerbate problems that exist in the office, as the furniture in use at home is rarely designed ergonomically.

Tech Neck

Your head weighs about five kilograms. This is equivalent to five bags of sugar, and is more than the average weight of a newborn baby! The cervical spine – the seven vertebrae of your neck – along with the muscles of your neck, are holding this weight. This requires a lot of work. If you are leaning forward, hunched over your computer, then you are creating a lot more work for your neck, leading to tension and fatigue.

Tech neck, or cervical kyphosis, is often the result. It is a phenomenon that has been becoming increasingly problematic in line with the rise of devices such as laptop computers and mobile phones. If you think about the position people adopt when they are on their digital devices, with their heads down and forward, it is easy to understand why this causes so many postural problems.

Poor posture not only causes physical pain, it also closes off the full capacity of the lungs, reducing your ability to take in air. For these reasons, it is important to pay attention to the ergonomics in your place of work.

In The Workplace - Office Ergonomics – Creating Your Ideal Set Up

Furniture

Desk

Ensure the space under your desk is clear, and that there is enough room for your legs under the desktop. If your desk is too low, raise the legs using blocks, making sure that the desk is completely stable. If your desk is too high then raise your chair.

Chair

It is important that your chair supports the natural curves of your spine. A chair with armrests provides support for your upper back and shoulders. Ensure your armrests are the correct height, so that your arms are supported with your shoulders in a relaxed position.

Footrest

If you cannot sit with your feet flat on the floor and your thighs parallel to the floor, use a footrest or stool in order to achieve this position.

Computer

Monitor

Positioned your monitor on the desk directly in front of your chair, at arm's length from your body. The top of the screen should be slightly below eye level.

Keyboard

Your keyboard should be directly in front of your monitor. Keep your hands below the level of your elbows, with your wrists straight. This creates a forty-five degree angle when you are typing. If you don't have a separate keyboard (and I highly recommend that you do) you run the risk of constantly looking down at your screen, which will create tension in your neck and upper back, thus closing off your breathing capacity.

Telephone

Use a headset or speaker to keep your hands free and ensure you are able to maintain a good posture.

In The Workplace - Top Tips

Standing Desk

A standing desk is a great option, as it keeps you really conscious of your posture, ensures you are using your core muscles, and gives you increased capacity to expand your lungs. Moving to a standing desk can take a bit of getting used to, but once you are over the initial oddity of it, you will no doubt become a convert.

Walking Meetings

Try to have one-on-one meetings with your colleagues walking outside. The fresh air, sunlight, and movement will boost your melatonin - which stabilizes the circadian rhythms of the body, and your oxytocin - which regulates your emotional responses and helps reduce stress. We all know that scientists have been telling us to move more during the day, so why not try this simple tip?

When making changes to your posture, you may need to play around adjusting heights and positions until you find the configuration that works perfectly for you. What you're looking to achieve is a position where your spine is comfortable, with your shoulders back, in order to ensure that your lungs can expand properly and the parasympathetic nervous system can engage, so that you are not in a perpetual state of anxiety.

Exercise – Cat/Cow Breathing

After 'downward dog', 'cat/cow' breathing is probably one of the first things you would learn about in any yoga class. You don't have to be a practicing yogi to get the powerful benefits of this simple spinal movement, which is paired with breath.

Place your hands and knees on the ground (if it's hard on your knees you can put a towel or cushion underneath them). The first motion is to inhale for a count of four as you scoop down in 'cow' in time with your breath. Your face will move up and your neck will be concave as you look up – don't strain your neck, only look up to the point that is comfortable for you. The shape your body is making is to have your belly dropped down and your spine in a 'U' shape for a count of four.

Pause briefly.

Gently exhale for a count of four as you scoop your back up into 'cat', so that your back looks like a dome, and your face is looking down, with your neck dropped.

Pause briefly.

Repeat this exercise for several rounds. Your spinal column and thoracic cavity will thank you for this.

If you don't want to do this in the workplace (but hey, who cares what others think?) then practice a few rounds of cat/cow breathing in the morning before you go to work.

If you are able to find a space at work, such as a breakout room, where you can go a couple of times during the day in order to do some cat/cow breathing, then this can really help you to realign your posture and become conscious of your breathing.

This is a great example of an easy balancing breathing technique, with the added benefit of spinal mobility.

Exercise – Hands Up

Raise your hands above your head, being careful to keep your shoulders down and back. Circle your left wrist with the fingers and thumb of your right hand, and then lean to the right, gently pulling your left arm, so that you are stretching out the side of your thoracic cavity and stretching the muscles along the side of your chest. This helps your chest to open up as you breathe from the diaphragm. Hold this position while you inhale and exhale for a count of four, then switch sides.

As you become more comfortable with this exercise, you can drop your hand to one side, as if leaning towards your thigh.

This is another great example of a balancing breathing technique that also helps keep your spine healthy and, additionally, stimulates the muscles required for easy twisting. It is also a great antidote to 'tech neck', and should be repeated regularly throughout the day. Why not start a trend with your co-workers?

Exercise – Neck

Follow the 'hands up' exercise with this simple neck exercise.

Gently put a little bit of hand weight on the left side of your head and drop your head to the right, breathing in for a count of four and out for a count of four. Whilst I am encouraging you to inhale deeply into your abdomen, I do like to concentrate my energy into my neck whilst carrying out this exercise, and particularly as I breathe out, I imagine a release. Your attention goes where your energy flows.

Switch sides and repeat.

Once you have done both sides, roll your head from left to right, breathing in for a count of four and out for a count of four. Change directions, so that you are rolling from right to left, while breathing in for a count of four and out for a count of four.

Seated in your chair, with your feet facing forwards, turn to the left and hold on to the back of your chair, so that you are twisting your body. Inhale for a count of four and exhale for a count of four, and then repeat on the other side.

Finally, roll your shoulders back and down while inhaling and exhaling for a count of four.

We are not designed to sit in front of a computer for hours at a time. Our attention span is approximately forty minutes, and so after this length of time it is important to have a little break. Carrying out these exercises as part of that break is extremely beneficial.

Exercise – Take The Floor

If you have the space and are able to step away from your desk, an additional stretch that you can perform is to lie on your back on the floor, with your knees up, and gently let them drop to the left, keeping your shoulders flat on the floor. Inhale for a count of four and exhale for a count of four, then repeat on the other side. This helps to give your spine some flexibility, which is extremely beneficial for your range of motion, and will help with your ability to twist. Being a 'four/four' breathing technique, this is also a balancing breath activity.

I want to emphasise that a lot of the stress and strain you place on your neck and shoulders stops you from breathing optimally. This can manifest as headaches, stiffness, and problems with your spine. By setting an alarm and taking the time to carry out one or more of these exercises every forty to sixty minutes, you can help to alleviate or avoid many of these problems.

As well as assisting with physical problems, by being mindful of your posture in the workplace you help to create another dimension to the feedback loop that ensures you attract more positive experiences into your working life.

In The Workplace - Case Study - Marco - Restricted Breathing

Marco came to me with concerns about how he was handling his workday. He was highly stressed and agitated, and not as productive as he would have liked to be. Marco had read somewhere that breathing properly could possibly help, so he approached me to see whether we could look at some basic breathing strategies that might contribute to his overall wellbeing.

We arranged to meet at his home office, so that I could observe him in his work environment. Like a lot of us, Marco carries a few extra kilos, and the first thing I noticed was that he was wearing a tight shirt, and pants that were also extremely tight. He was, however, highly fashionable – lol!

These tight 'fashionable' clothes were restricting his abdomen. As a result, he was breathing from his upper chest, to the extent that his shoulders were moving quite markedly, and yet his diaphragm was almost frozen. I asked him if he had neck and shoulder pain, and he said that his neck and shoulders were constantly sore.

Breathing using ancillary muscles quite often causes neck and shoulder pain, because you're generating thousands of movements in your neck and shoulders every day and millions every year, and it's simply not the way your body was designed to work.

I asked Marco to sit at his desk and work on his computer, as he would normally work. He had a really great, ergonomically designed chair, but he sat in the chair with his butt right at the edge of the seat, which forced his back into a C-shaped curve.

I watched him as he typed out an email. He was hunched over, breathing from his upper body, his neck was at the wrong angle, and his computer screen was too low for him. It was clear to see that if he was doing that all day, every day, he would feel constantly stressed.

After a few minutes, I asked if I could take his place in the chair. I sat down and rearranged things a little bit, so that his monitor was at eye-level and his arms would be at a forty-five degree angle when he was using his mouse and his keyboard. I sat with my butt against the back of the seat, and my spine upright, in a natural S bend.

I then asked him to try it out for himself. He tried the position, and his posture was great, but he still wasn't breathing from his abdomen. He just didn't know how to breathe diaphragmatically.

I invited him to place his hand a couple of centimetres in front of his belly and asked him to breathe out so that his belly touched his hand. He had spent so many years training his body to breathe in the wrong way that he couldn't do it.

The best way to create breath awareness in this situation is to lie on the floor. In this position, it is a lot easier to be conscious of your breathing apparatus.

Marco then lay on the floor. In order to carry out the exercise properly he needed to unbuckle his pants, which just goes to show how tight they were. Instantly, his stomach popped out and his abdomen began to move slightly. I then asked him to place his left hand on his stomach and his right hand in the middle of his chest, and inhale through his nose for four slow counts, imagining that he was breathing to a place below his navel, almost as if he was filling a balloon up from the bottom, and then to breathe out through his nose for four slow counts, as if he was emptying the balloon from the top down.

The goal of this exercise is to breathe without your chest moving. After you've done a few rounds of this exercise, you really get an idea about whether your chest is moving or not.

Marco quickly found that he was breathing deeply from his diaphragm, and was really quite surprised by this. He felt very comfortable and free, and realised that his pants and his shirt were far too tight for his body, and that they were restricting his breathing.

He confided in me that he was embarrassed

that he had put on a lot of weight, and he didn't want to show his big stomach. I explained that the reality was his diaphragm wasn't working properly, which meant he wasn't digesting his food properly, and his abdominal muscles weren't working in the way that they were designed to work. This meant he wasn't going to get any muscle definition, because the constant state of stress that his abs were in would make them weaker (it's counter-intuitive – people hold their stomachs in, thinking it will give them muscle definition, when in reality if you don't use your abdomen properly you're never going to get muscle definition).

I then placed a relatively heavy book, weighing a couple of kilos, over his navel. Again, I asked him to inhale through his nose for four slow counts, and then exhale through his nose for four slow counts, consciously moving the book up and down, without moving his shoulders and upper chest. This creates a heightened awareness of breathing from the abdomen rather than from the chest.

These exercises are very useful, because once you learn to breathe in the way you're designed to breathe, it is far easier to replicate the technique in your day-to-day life.

Finally, still lying on his back, I asked Marco to carry out a 'compartment breathing' exercise, which is a three-count, three-phase breath, designed to create an awareness of the different muscles used in breathing.

Compartment breathing is almost like you're filling up three chambers. On each breath, you inhale deeply through your nose. With the first breath, you take your attention to your lower abdomen, allowing yourself to feel the rise of your belly. On the second breath, you take your attention to your intercostal muscles, allowing yourself to feel the expansion of your ribcage. Try and imagine expansion is happening 360 degrees around your ribcage. On the third breath, you take the attention to your accessory muscles, which are located in your upper chest, and are the muscles that do not take a primary role in your breathing. These are the muscles that you use if you have been running and you're gasping for air once you stop. Allow yourself to feel the slight movement of your neck, shoulders, and back.

After about ten minutes of doing those three exercises, Marco had a really great idea of where he should be breathing. He buckled his pants, got up, and sat back down at his computer.

Once again, even though he knew where he needed to breathe from, he found it challenging, because his clothes were physically constraining him. At this point, he realised that vanity had to go out the window, and his pants and shirt needed to go up a size or two. However, by now, he understood that this was a positive thing, as he recognised it was going to reduce his stress levels.

Over the next couple of weeks, he practiced his three supine breathing exercises. When he was sitting vertically at his desk, he started to imagine his diaphragm was expanding, his abdomen was expanding, and that inhaling was a fluid motion.

We met again four weeks later, and Marco reported that he was feeling absolutely amazing. He'd bought larger pants and felt much more comfortable and far less stressed. His back and shoulders were no longer constantly sore, and he had found that he was able to sit at his desk for long periods of time and have conversations on the phone and online, in a way he had not been able to do before.

By becoming breath aware, and understanding how his body was designed to breathe, Marco was able to free himself from many of the problems associated with his poor breath and posture.

Three months later, Marco was still using these exercises and had lost several kilos, which he put down to a reduction in stress and feeling generally better about himself and his work environment.

Key Takeaways

- Designing how you work has an impact on how you feel throughout your work day.
- Clothes can restrict how you breathe and have an impact on your posture.
- When your body is reminded how it naturally operates, it quickly adjusts.

Chapter Nine

Laughter Yoga

Several years ago, my business was in a not a great position. My business partner and I had very different expectations. She was close to retirement, and I was planning to continue with the company for a number of years. As a result, we were disconnected about the way in which we wanted to take the business forward. I was getting very stressed and agitated about it. I'd stopped meditating, and I hadn't been introduced to the concept of conscious breathing, so I didn't have many clear strategies to manage the stress I was experiencing.

When we are really stressed and anxious, the body can react. Some of us hear the messages the body is sending us, and some of us don't. If we don't hear the messages, the body can start sending increasingly loud messages.

In order to get away from the troubles I was having with my business, my life partner and I decided to visit Colombia, Peru, and Ecuador. It was the trip of a lifetime, and I was really excited and looking forward to getting away from the stress of everything.

We were flying from America to Columbia, and during the flight the cabin crew served us a meal. I was trying to eat, but the food was falling out of my mouth. I couldn't work out what was happening. The side of my face was going numb, and it was really distressing. My partner has a medical background, and said that it seemed as though I was experiencing Bell's palsy, or idiopathic facial palsy, which is a condition where your facial muscles freeze, and you have a partial paralysis of your face.

We arrived in Bogota in the middle of night, by which time I was experiencing full palsy down one side of my face. First thing the next morning, we went to a large hospital in the centre of Bogota, which isn't the way anyone wants to start an international holiday. A busy Bogota hospital on a Sunday morning is quite an experience, and one I wouldn't recommend for anyone's bucket list.

Once we got past the security guards with machine guns, we used a combination of Spanglish and Google to explain to the nurses what was going on. I was finally seen by a doctor who spoke a little bit of English, I was diagnosed, given an eye-patch and a prescription for the drugs I needed, and I was able to enjoy the rest of my holiday, in a slightly more piratical way than I had planned.

When recovering from Bell's palsy, the doctors and physiotherapists advise you to exercise your facial muscles to avoid permanent paralysis.

Many of these exercises involve smiling, and I discovered that the more I practised smiling, the better I started to feel. I thought back to my psychology degree, and everything I had learned about the body/brain feedback loop. I realised that this is what I was experiencing. My brain could not tell the difference between smiling to exercise my facial muscles (I call this 'fake smiling') and smiling because I was happy. This is because if your body is carrying out an action, your brain thinks it is motivated by an experience. This is the reality of 'fake it till you make it'.

Of course, when people are very depressed, it's really hard to do this. But it does make a massive difference. The more I researched this phenomenon, the more interested I became. In the course of my research, I came across an article on laughter yoga.

Laughter yoga was started in India in 1995, by Doctor Madan Kataria. Dr Kataria was an allopathic physician, looking at ways to improve recovery times for his patients. He thought about the concept that laughter is the best medicine, and the practice of laughter yoga grew from there.

There are some yogic exercises and pranayama breathing exercises involved in laughter yoga, and he extended these traditional practices by adding exercises that simulate and stimulate laughter. Since 1995, laughter yoga has grown to become a worldwide movement.

I joined a Melbourne laughter club, and I absolutely loved it. Within a year, I had become a fully qualified laughter yoga instructor. Many people don't understand how you can 'learn how to laugh', as it is something that we think of as coming naturally, but laughter yoga is a very structured process that helps people to laugh in a sustained way, as the greatest benefits come with laughing for about twenty minutes. The laughter yoga program takes you through warm-up exercises and themed laughter exercises, and gives you the ability to laugh for no reason whatsoever.

For many adults, the sheer joy of laughter is replaced by the business of being busy. Children laugh uncontrollably, having a whale of a time for no reason. But adults often suppress laughter. In some cultures, people laugh with their hand over their mouth, because they don't want to be seen to be laughing.

The ability to experience pure joy can affect our whole way of being. Research shows that laughter can positively change outcomes for people with medical conditions, and can even assist with weight loss[2]. Laughter is proven to increase dopamine, melatonin,

[2]Bast ES, Berry EM. Laugh Away the Fat? Therapeutic Humor in the Control of Stress-induced Emotional Eating. Rambam Maimonides Med J. 2014 Jan 21;5(1):e0007. doi: 10.5041/RMMJ.10141. PMID: 24498514; PMCID: PMC3904482.

and serotonin[3], and is also a really great way to really connect with your diaphragm. A lot of people who breathe from their chests find that laughter really helps them to discover their diaphragm.

I really encourage people to go to a laughter club in order to learn how to start laughing for no reason. I like to laugh in the shower, as part of my daily conscious breathing. Laughing in the shower is something that you can easily fit it into your existing morning routine. The physical act of laughing is an energising breath, because you're increasing the rate of your breathing.

A lot of workplaces bring laughter yoga instructors in to help improve the health and wellbeing of their teams. It's a really fantastic team building activity - the company that laughs together lasts together!

Bringing laughter into the workplace is extremely beneficial. You don't need a formal laughter yoga club, you can laugh for no reason at all. Many

[3]Yim J. Therapeutic Benefits of Laughter in Mental Health: A Theoretical Review. Tohoku J Exp Med. 2016 Jul;239(3):243-9. doi: 10.1620/tjem.239.243. PMID: 27439375.

workplaces have laughter circles, where they come together and just laugh. Imagine the joy of just laughing with your workmates for a couple of minutes every day!

Laughing in the workplace not only improves physical and mental wellbeing, it also breaks down hierarchies. You can be the CEO or the work experience kid - everyone's equal in a laughter environment. Laughter is a massive equaliser.

Happiness and joy are infectious, and so, from a leadership perspective, laughter is a really great way of raising the energy of your team, connecting your team to each other, and bringing conscious breathing into the workplace.

Key Takeaways

- The body/brain feedback loop cannot tell the difference between fake and real emotions, so there is a sensation of happiness even if you manufacture the emotion.
- Laughing is a great way to activate your diaphragm.
- Laughing (in the shower) once a day will lift your mood.
- Laughter in the workplace is a great team-building activity.

Conclusion

Understanding the intuitive nature of being in touch with your breath, the importance of connecting to your breath, and how to access this connection through simple exercises, enables you to incorporate conscious breathing into your life. If you are now able to stop and take stock even just a couple of times a day in order to breathe deeply, then this book will have served its purpose.

Sometimes the simplest things have the biggest impact. We are born knowing how to breathe, but as we go through life we disconnect from our essential nature. It's this disconnection that creates the discomfort that many of us face on a day-to-day basis. We look for all sorts of ways to fix this disconnection, when the answer is really simple. By just stopping, taking a breath, and being in the moment when you breathe fully, you can re-establish the connection to your essential nature.

Conscious breathing is a tool that we have with us all the time, but because of its simplicity, many people don't recognise or utilise it. Now, having developed your understanding, you can start to bring the benefits of conscious breathing into every aspect of your life.

If you're a businessperson looking for a coach, contact Braith. Braith can tailor coaching for specific desired outcomes or work with you on an eight-week results programme.

Contact Braith directly at:
https://braithbamkin.com.au/

Braith Bamkin

Author Biography

Braith has been a business owner for many years. In spite of commercial success, he always had a strong sense that something was missing.

After experiencing a period of extreme stress and anxiety, with physical symptoms that culminated in the facial paralysis Bell's palsy, Braith recognised that he needed to find the missing piece, although he still wasn't sure how.

While carrying out facial exercises to overcome Bell's palsy, which included practicing smiling, Braith found that his stress and anxiety began to decrease. Thinking back to his psychology degree, Braith recognised that this was Behavioural Activation Theory, more commonly known as 'fake it till you make it'. Essentially, his brain couldn't tell the difference between smiling as an exercise, and smiling because he was happy.

From here, Braith began to explore the concepts of laughter yoga and conscious breathing, and became a certified instructor in both practices.

Braith's interest in the ability to increase feelings of wellbeing, and to change our energetic state from negative to positive through Behavioural Activation Theory, continued to grow.

As a long-term yoga practitioner, he saw clear connections between the yogic breathing technique 'pranayama', conscious breathing, laughter yoga, and Behavioural Activation Theory.

Braith recognised that many aspects of pranayama and modern Western breath work teaching were overly complicated. As a result, they remained largely inaccessible to many people.

And so *Breathe Easy: Simple Ways to Stay Well Connected* was born. By combining his knowledge of business, psychology, laughter, pranayama, and conscious breathing, to create a simple and accessible way for professionals to reduce their stress, increase their wellbeing, and reconnect with themselves and others in a positive and beneficial way, Braith has created a system of conscious breathing that is easily applied in both a professional and personal context.